The Ultimate Keto Vegan Cookbook Recipes

Healthy and delicious keto vegan recipes

Nancy Graham

Please consult a licensed professional before attempting any techniques outlined in this book.

By reading this document, the reader agrees that under no circumstances is the author responsible for any losses, direct or indirect, which are incurred as a result of the use of information contained within this document, including, but not limited to, — errors, omissions, or inaccuracies.

TABLE OF CONTENTS

Berry Acai Breakfast Smoothie

Preparation Time: 2 Minutes - Cooking Time: 0 Minutes - Servings: 1

Ingredients:

- 1 cup Silk Tofu
- 2 tbsp. Coconut Cream
- 1 cup Ice Cubes
- ¼ cup Raspberries
- 2 tbsp. Acai Powder
- 3 tbsp. Soy Protein Powder(Vanilla-flavored)

Directions:

1. Combine all ingredients in a blender.
2. Blend until smooth.

Nutrition: Calories: 266 / Fat: 20 g / Protein: 18 g / Carbs: 10 g

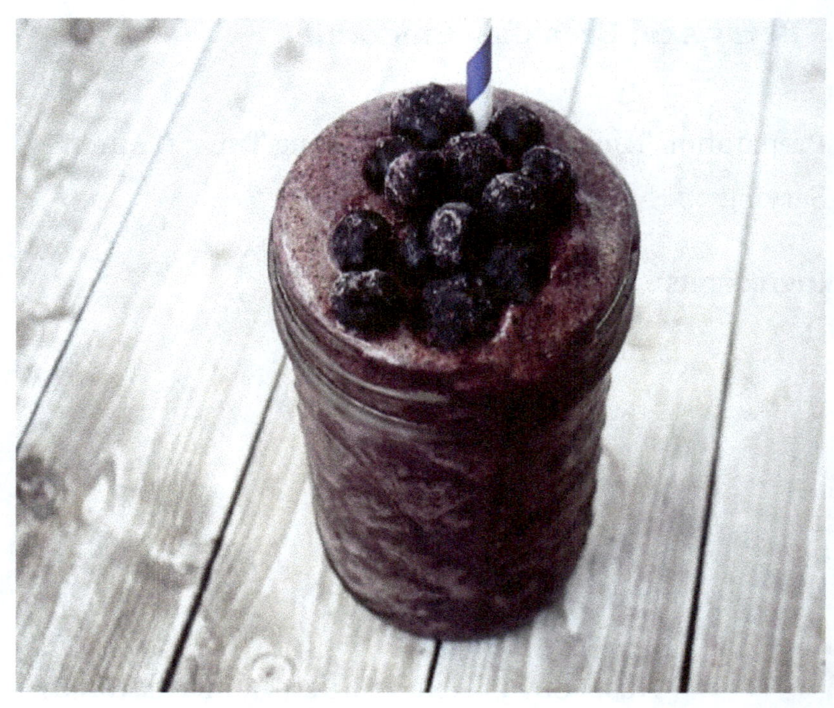

Keto Choco "Oats"

Preparation Time: 5 minutes - Cooking Time: 5 minutes - Servings: 2

Ingredients:

- 200 g Cauliflower, riced
- 1 cup Coconut Milk
- 2 tbsp. Flax Seeds
- 1 tbsp. Erythritol
- 2 tbsp. Cocoa Powder
- 1 tbsp. Vanilla Extract
- 50 g fresh Raspberries
- 1 tbsp. Cacao Nibs

Directions:

1. Combine cauliflower, coconut milk, flax seeds, erythritol, cocoa powder, and vanilla extract in a pot.
2. Simmer for 3-5 minutes.
3. Ladle into bowls and top with fresh raspberries and cacao nibs.

Nutrition: Calories: 464 / Fat: 41 g / Protein: 22 g / Carbs: 10 g

Banana Hazelnut Waffles

Preparation Time: 3 minutes - Cooking Time: 5 minutes - Servings: 2

Ingredients:

- 2 tbsp. Flaxseed Meal
- 1/2 cup Almond Flour
- 2 tbsp. Erythritol
- 1 tsp Baking Powder
- 1 tsp Ground Cinnamon
- 2 tbsp. Hazelnut Butter
- ½ cup Coconut Milk
- 1 tsp Banana Essence

Directions:

1. Process all ingredients in a blender until smooth.
2. Pour into waffle iron and cook for 3-5 minutes.

Nutrition: Calories: 316 / Fat: 31 g / Protein: 3 g / Carbs: 9 g

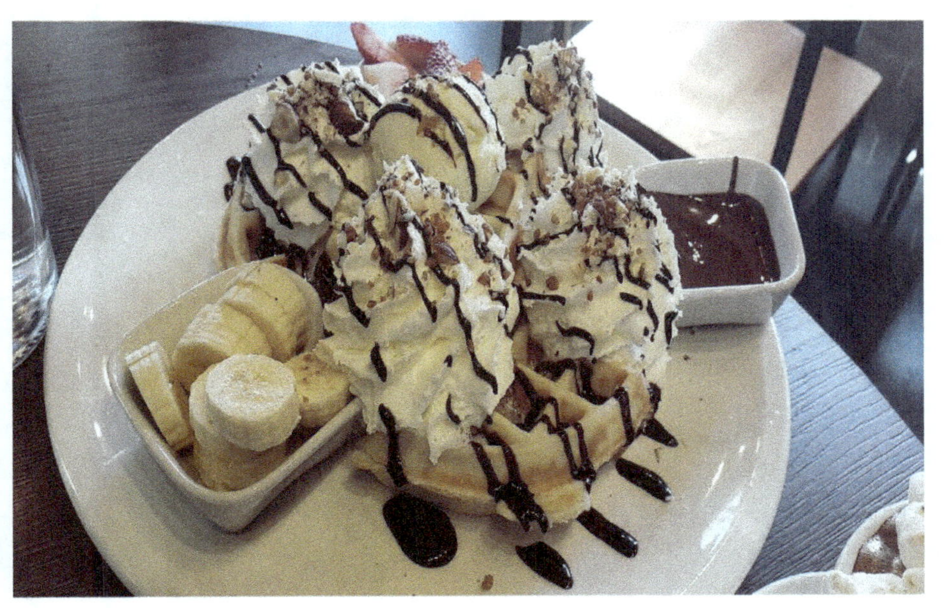

Vegan Breakfast Skillet

Preparation Time: 3 minutes - Cooking Time: 5 minutes
Servings: 4

Ingredients:

- 3 tbsp. Olive Oil
- 400 g Firm Tofu, drained and crumbled
- 20 g Chickpeas
- 100 g Spinach
- 1 tbsp. Garlic Powder
- 1 tsp Paprika
- ½ tsp Turmeric Powder
- ¼ tsp Salt
- ¼ tsp Pepper

Directions:

1. Heat olive oil in a skillet.
2. Add crumbled tofu and stir for 2-3 minutes.
3. Stir in all the spices.
4. Add chickpeas and spinach — sauté for another minute.
5. Serve hot.

Nutrition: Calories: 271 / Fat: 19 g / Protein: 18 g / Carbs: 10 g

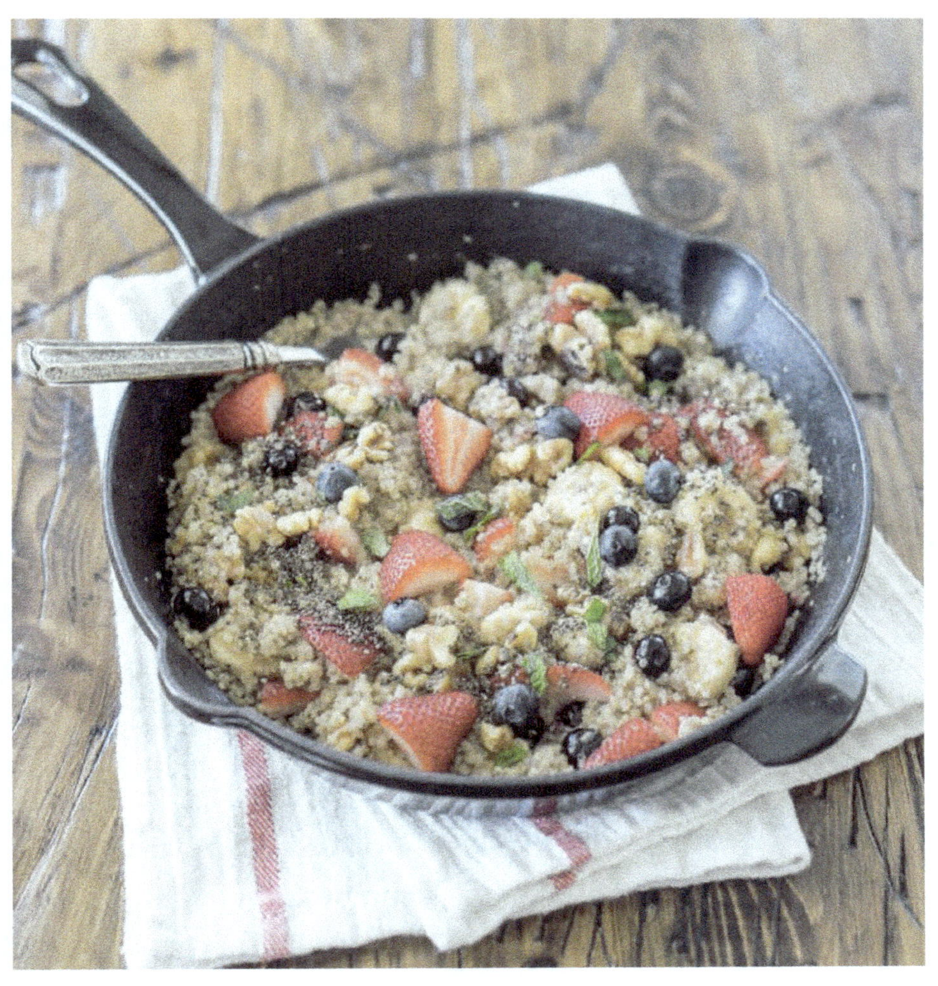

Vegan Breakfast Hash

Preparation Time: 15 minutes - Cooking Time: 5 minutes - Servings: 4

Ingredients:

- 1 cup Cooked Quinoa
- 1 cup Shredded Broccoli
- 2 tbsp. Flax Seed
- ½ cup Coconut Flour
- 1 tsp Garlic Powder
- 1 tsp Onion Powder
- 2 tbsp. Coconut Oil

Directions:

1. Stir flax seeds with half a cup of water in a large mixing bowl. Leave for a few minutes.
2. Stir in all remaining ingredients.
3. From the mixture into patties.
4. Heat vegetable oil in a pan.
5. Fry the patties for 2-3 minutes per side.

Nutrition: Calories: 135 / Fat: 10 g / Protein: 3 g / Carbs: 10 g

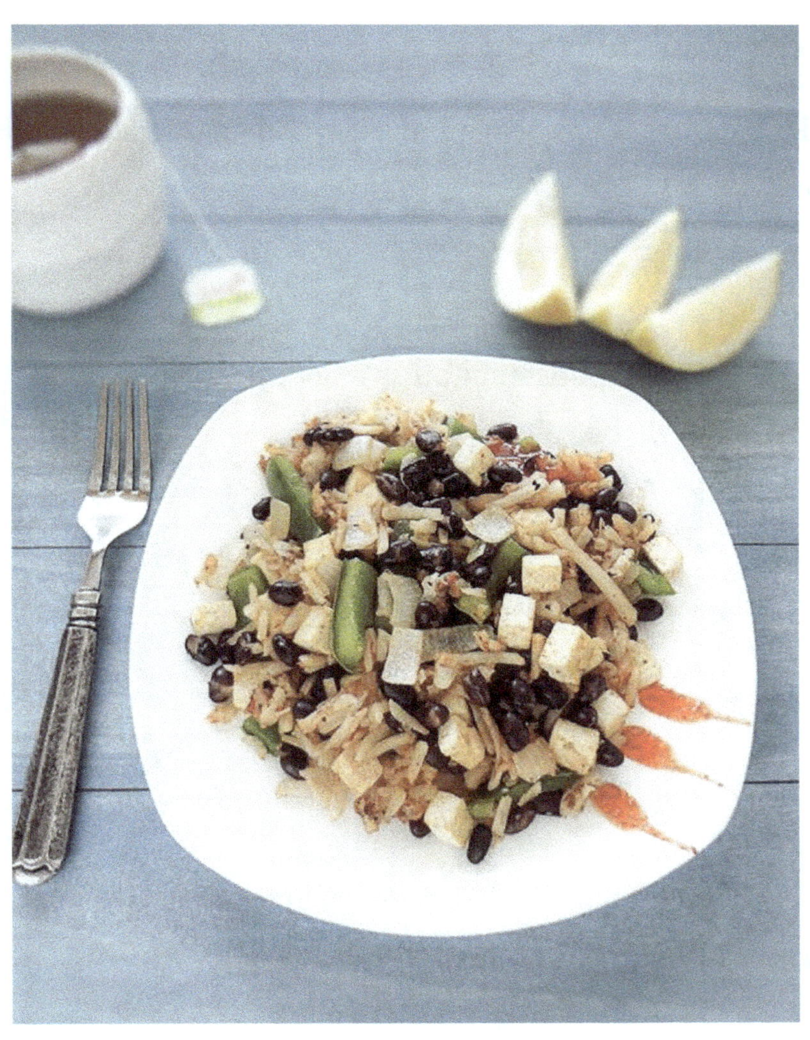

Tiramisu Chia Pudding

Preparation Time: 15 minutes - Cooking Time: 5 minutes - Servings: 1

Ingredients:

- 1/4 cup Chia Seeds
- 2 tsp Instant Coffee
- 2 tbsp. Coconut Cream
- ¾ cup Water
- 1 tbsp. Erythritol
- 1 tsp Powdered Cinnamon

Directions:

1. Combine all ingredients in a mason jar.
2. Shake until well blended.
3. Chill for at least 20 minutes.

Nutrition: Calories: 112 / Fat: 9 g / Protein: 3 g / Carbs: 9 g

Tofu and Spinach Frittata

Preparation Time: 15 minutes - Cooking Time: 5 minutes - Servings: 4

Ingredients:

- 400 g Firm Tofu
- 2 tbsp. tamari
- 2 tbsp. Nutritional Yeast
- 1 tsp Turmeric
- 1 tbsp. Garlic Powder
- 2 cups Baby Spinach, chopped
- 1 Red Bell Pepper, chopped
- 2 tbsp. Olive Oil

Directions:

1. Combine tofu, tamari, nutritional yeast, turmeric, and garlic powder in a food processor. Blend until smooth.
2. Fold in the spinach and bell pepper into the mixture.
3. Brush an iron skillet with olive oil.
4. Pour the mixture into the skillet.
5. Bake for 25 minutes at 360F.

Nutrition: Calories: 236 / Fat: 16 g / Protein: 18 g / Carbs: 9 g

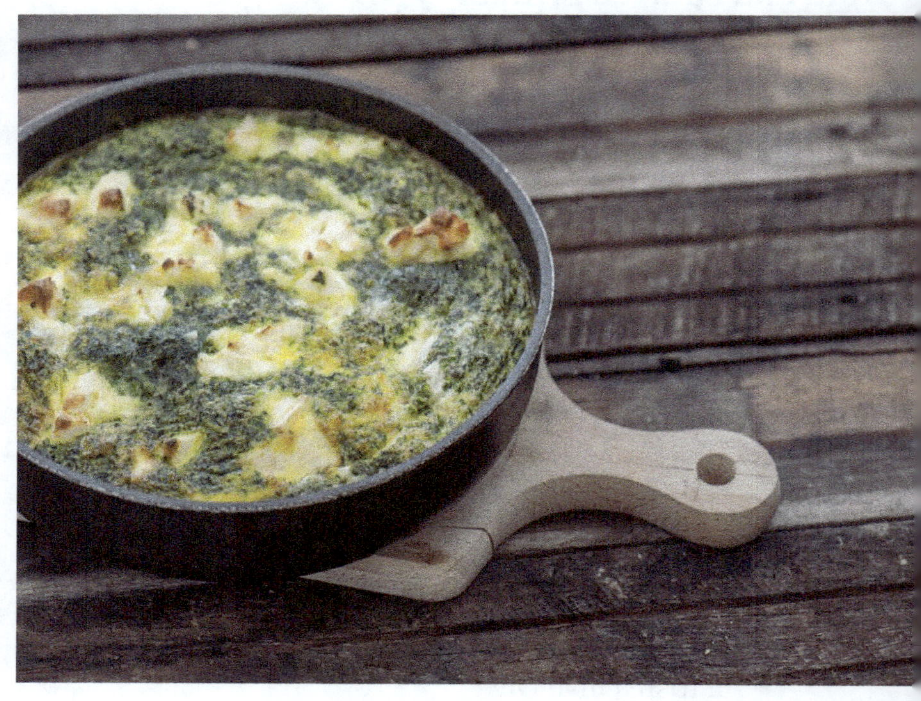

Fat-Bomb Frappuccino

Preparation Time: 15 minutes - Cooking Time: 5 minutes - Servings: 1

Ingredients:

- 2/3 cup Brewed Coffee
- ¼ cup Almond Milk
- 2 tbsp. Erythritol
- 1 tsp Vanilla Extract
- 2 tbsp. Coconut Oil
- ½ cup Ice Cubes

Directions:

1. Mix all ingredients in a blender until smooth.

Nutrition: Calories: 278 / Fat: 28 g / Protein: 1 g / Carbs: 6 g

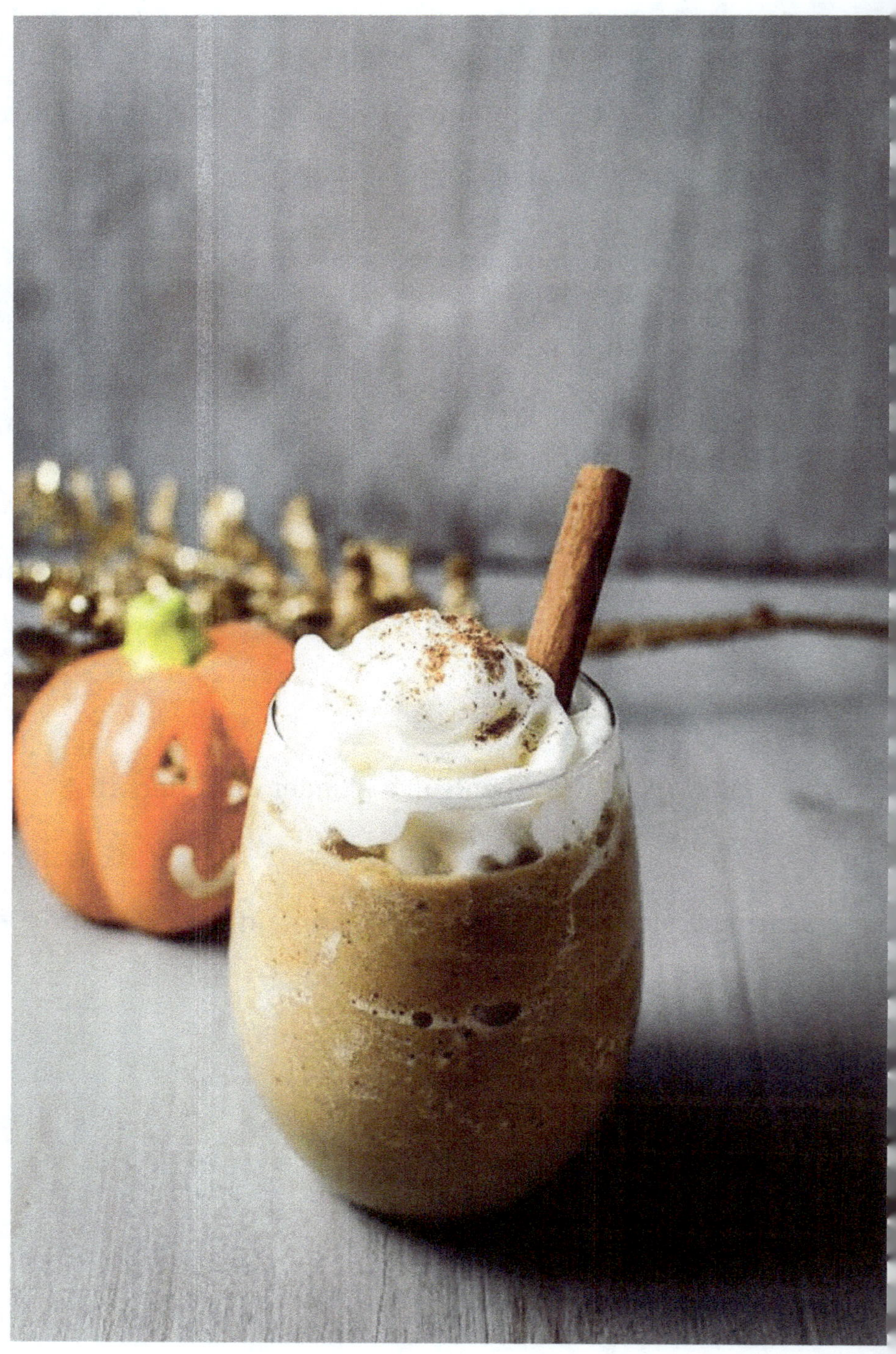

Almond Hemp Heart Porridge

Preparation Time: 10 minutes - Cooking Time: 2 minutes - Servings: 2

Ingredients:

- ¼ cup almond flour
- ½ tsp cinnamon
- ¾ tsp vanilla extract
- 5 drops stevia
- 1 tbsp. chia seeds
- 2 tbsp. ground flax seed
- ½ cup hemp hearts
- 1 cup unsweetened coconut milk

Directions:

1. Add all ingredients except almond flour to a saucepan. Stir to combine.
2. Heat over medium heat until it starts to boil lightly.
3. Once start bubbling, then stir well and cook for 1 minute more.
4. Remove from heat and stir in almond flour.
5. Serve immediately and enjoy it.

Nutrition: Calories 329 / Fat 24.4 g / Carbohydrates 9.2 g / Sugar 1.8 g / Protein 16.2 g

Cholesterol 0 mg

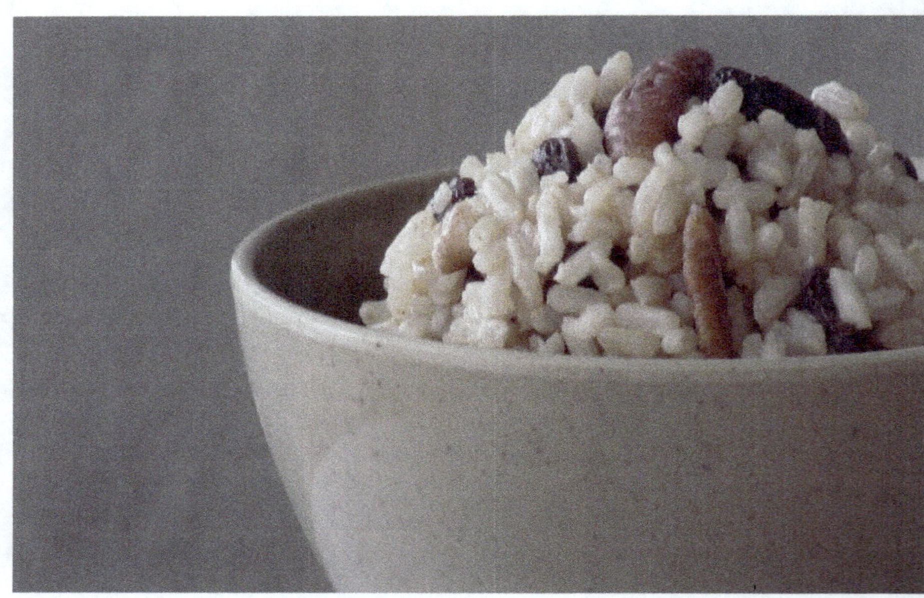

Chocolate Strawberry Milkshake

Preparation Time: 5 minutes - Cooking Time: 0 minutes - Servings: 2

Ingredients:

- 1 cup of ice cubes
- ¼ cup unsweetened cocoa powder
- 2 scoops vegan protein powder
- 1 cup strawberries
- 2 cups unsweetened coconut milk

Directions:

1. Add all ingredients into the blender and blend until smooth and creamy.
2. Serve immediately and enjoy it.

Nutrition: Calories 221 / Fat 5.7 g / Carbohydrates 15 g / Sugar 6.8 g / Protein 27.7 g

Cholesterol 0 mg

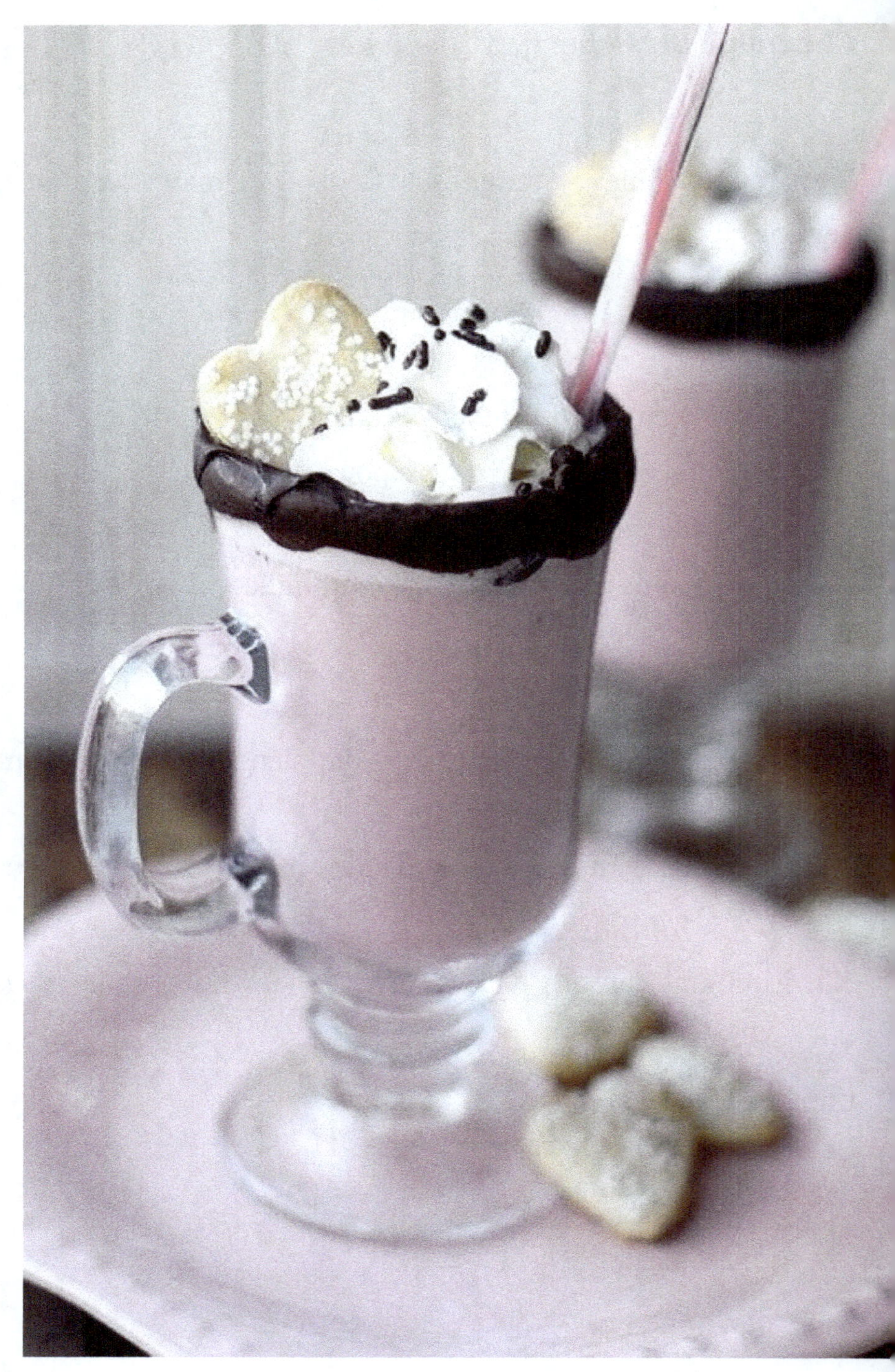

Chia Cinnamon Smoothie

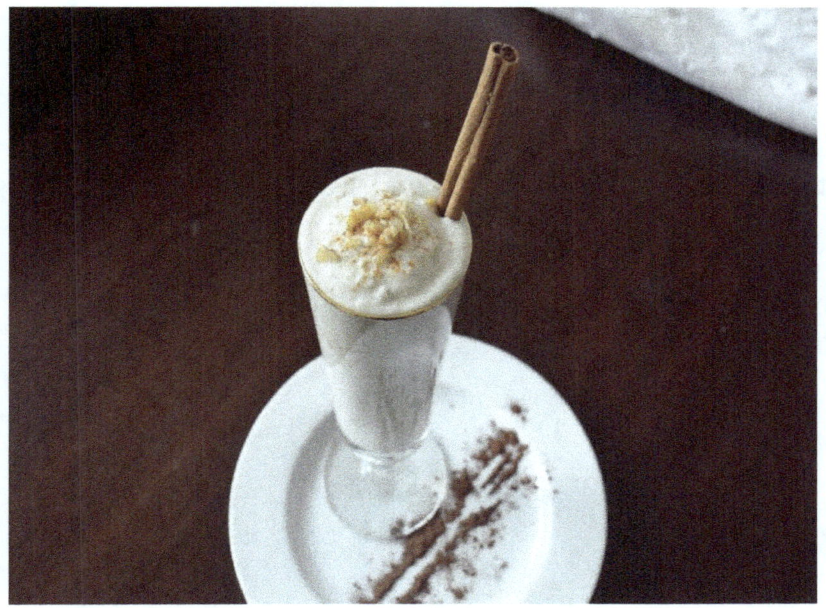

Preparation Time: 5 minutes - Cooking Time: 0 minutes - Servings: 1

Ingredients:

- 2 scoops vanilla protein powder
- 1 tbsp. chia seeds
- ½ tsp cinnamon
- 1 tbsp. coconut oil
- ½ cup of water
- ½ cup unsweetened coconut milk

Directions:

1. Add all ingredients into the blender and blend until smooth and creamy.
2. Serve immediately and enjoy it.

Nutrition: Calories 397 / Fat 23.9 g / Carbohydrates 13.4 g / Sugar 0 g / Protein 31.6 g

Cholesterol 0 mg

Vegetable Tofu Scramble

Preparation Time: 20 minutes - Cooking Time: 5 minutes - Servings: 2

Ingredients:

- 1 block firm tofu, drained and crumbled
- ½ tsp turmeric - ¼ tsp garlic powder
- 1 cup spinach - 1 red pepper, chopped
- 10 oz. mushrooms, chopped
- ½ onion, chopped - 1 tbsp. olive oil
- Pepper - Salt

Directions:

1. Heat olive oil in a large pan over medium heat.
2. Add onion, pepper, and mushrooms and sauté until cooked.
3. Add crumbled tofu, spices, and spinach. Stir well and cook for 3-5 minutes.
4. Serve and enjoy.

Nutrition: Calories 159 / Fat 9.6 g / Carbohydrates 13.7 g / Sugar 7 g / Protein 9.6 g

Cholesterol 0 mg

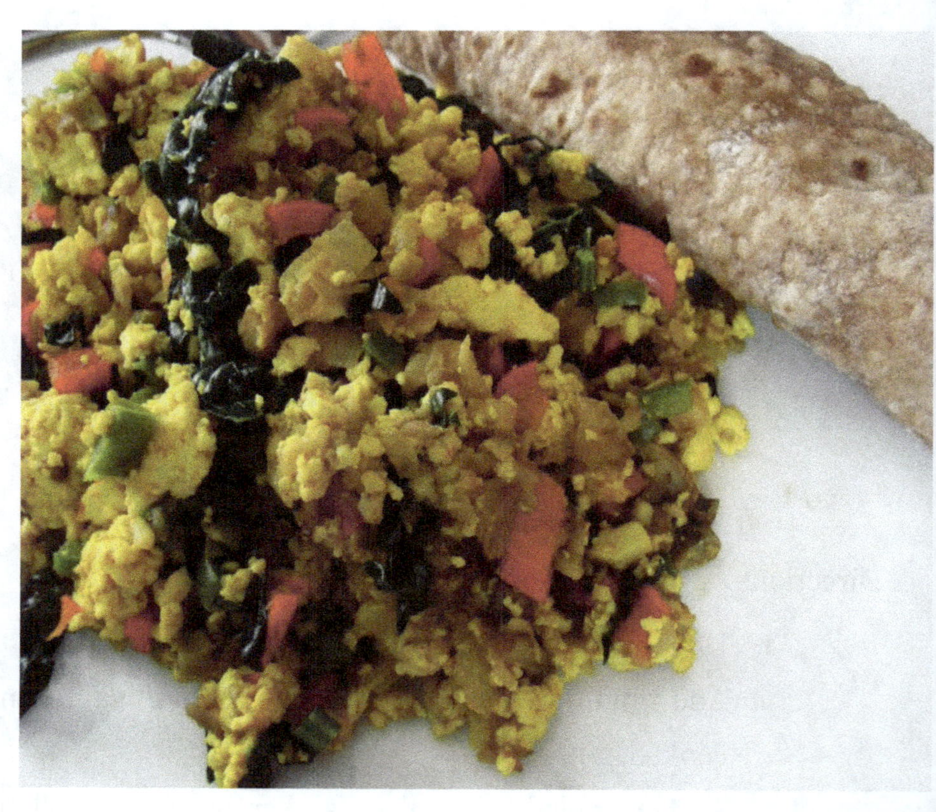

Breakfast Granola

Preparation Time: 30 minutes - Cooking Time: 23 minutes - Servings: 15

Ingredients:

- 1 tsp ground ginger - 1 tsp ground cinnamon
- ¼ cups coconut oil, melted - 1 cup walnuts, chopped
- 2/3 cup pumpkin seeds - 2/3 cup sunflower seeds
- ½ cup flaxseeds - 3 cups desiccated coconut

Directions:

1. Add all ingredients into the large bowl and toss well.
2. Spread the granola mixture on a baking tray and bake at 350 F/ 180 C for 20 minutes. Turn granola mixture with a spoon after every 3 minutes.
3. Allow to cool completely and serve.

Nutrition: Calories 208 / Fat 17 g / Carbohydrates 11.4 g / Sugar 5.8 g / Protein 4.1 g

Cholesterol 0 mg

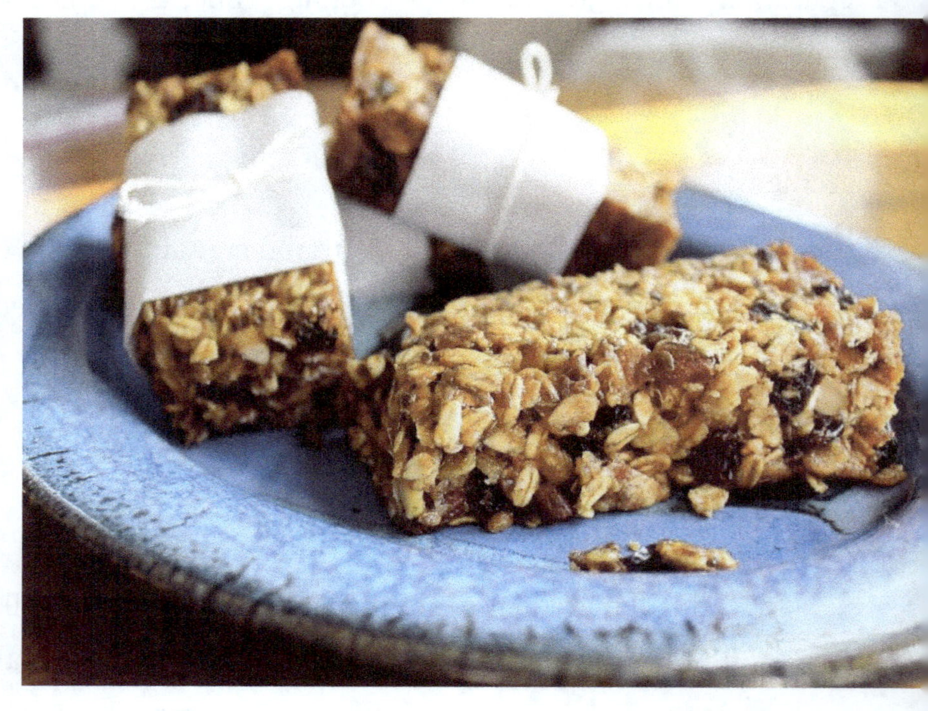

Grain-Free Overnight Oats

Preparation Time: 10 minutes - Cooking Time: 0 minutes - Servings: 1

Ingredients:

- 2/3 cup unsweetened coconut milk
- 2 tsp chia seeds
- 2 tbsp. vanilla protein powder
- ½ tbsp. coconut flour
- 3 tbsp. hemp hearts

Directions:

1. Add all ingredients into the glass jar and stir to combine.
2. Close jar with lid and place in the refrigerator overnight.
3. Top with fresh berries and serve.

Nutrition: Calories 378 / Fat 22.5 g / Carbohydrates 15 g / Sugar 1.5 g / Protein 27 g

Cholesterol 0 mg

Almond Coconut Porridge

Preparation Time: 10 minutes - Cooking Time: 2 minutes - Servings: 2

Ingredients:

- ¾ cup unsweetened almond milk
- ½ tsp vanilla extract
- 1 ½ tbsp. ground flaxseed
- 3 tbsp. ground almonds
- 6 tbsp. unsweetened shredded coconut
- Pinch of sea salt

Directions:

1. Add almond milk in microwave-safe bowl and microwave for 2 minutes.
2. Add remaining ingredients and stir well and cook for 1 minute.
3. Top with fresh berries and serve.

Nutrition: Calories 197 / Fat 17.4 g / Carbohydrates 8.3 g / Sugar 0.6 g / Protein 4.2 g

Cholesterol 0 mg

Avocado Chocó Cinnamon Smoothie

Preparation Time: 5 minutes - Cooking Time: 0 minutes - Servings: 1

Ingredients:

- ½ tsp coconut oil
- 5 drops liquid stevia
- ¼ tsp vanilla extract
- 1 tsp ground cinnamon
- 2 tsp unsweetened cocoa powder
- ½ avocado
- ¾ cup unsweetened coconut milk

Directions:

1. Add all ingredients into the blender and blend until smooth and creamy.
2. Serve immediately and enjoy it.

Nutrition: Calories 95 / Fat 8.3 g / Carbohydrates 5.1 g / Sugar 0.2 g / Protein 1.2 g

Cholesterol 0 mg

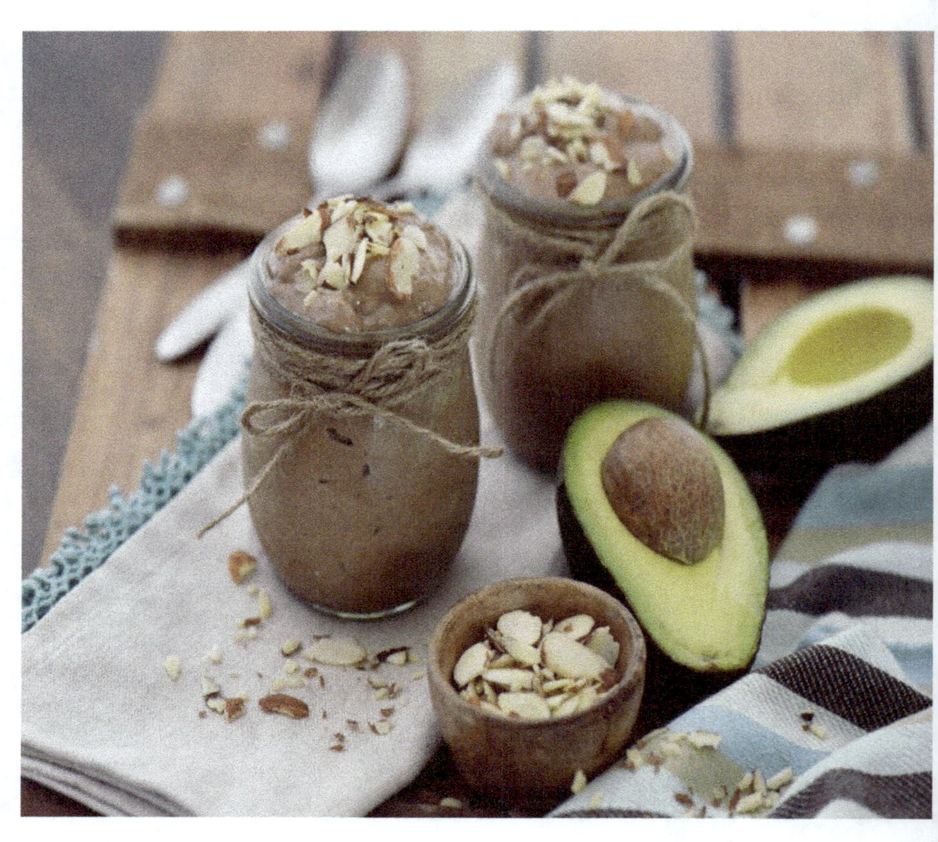

Strawberry Chia Matcha Pudding

Preparation Time: 10 minutes - Cooking Time: 0 minutes - Servings: 1

Ingredients:

- 5 drops liquid stevia
- 2 strawberries, diced
- 1 ½ tbsp. chia seeds
- ¾ cup unsweetened coconut milk
- ½ tsp matcha powder

Directions:

1. Add all ingredients except strawberries into the glass jar and mix well.
2. Close jar with lid and place in the refrigerator for 4 hours.
3. Add strawberries into the pudding and mix well.
4. Serve and enjoy.

Nutrition: Calories 93 / Fat 6.5 g / Carbohydrates 5.6 g / Sugar 1.2 g / Protein 2.5 g

Cholesterol 0 mg

Avocado Breakfast Smoothie

Preparation Time: 5 minutes - Cooking Time: 0 minutes
Servings: 2

Ingredients:

- 5 drops liquid stevia
- ¼ cup of ice cubes
- ½ avocado
- 1 tsp vanilla extract
- 1 cup unsweetened coconut milk

Directions:

1. Add all ingredients into the blender and blend until smooth and creamy.
2. Serve immediately and enjoy it.

Nutrition: Calories 131 / Fat 11.8 g / Carbohydrates 5.6 g / Sugar 0.5 g / Protein 1 g

Cholesterol 0 mg

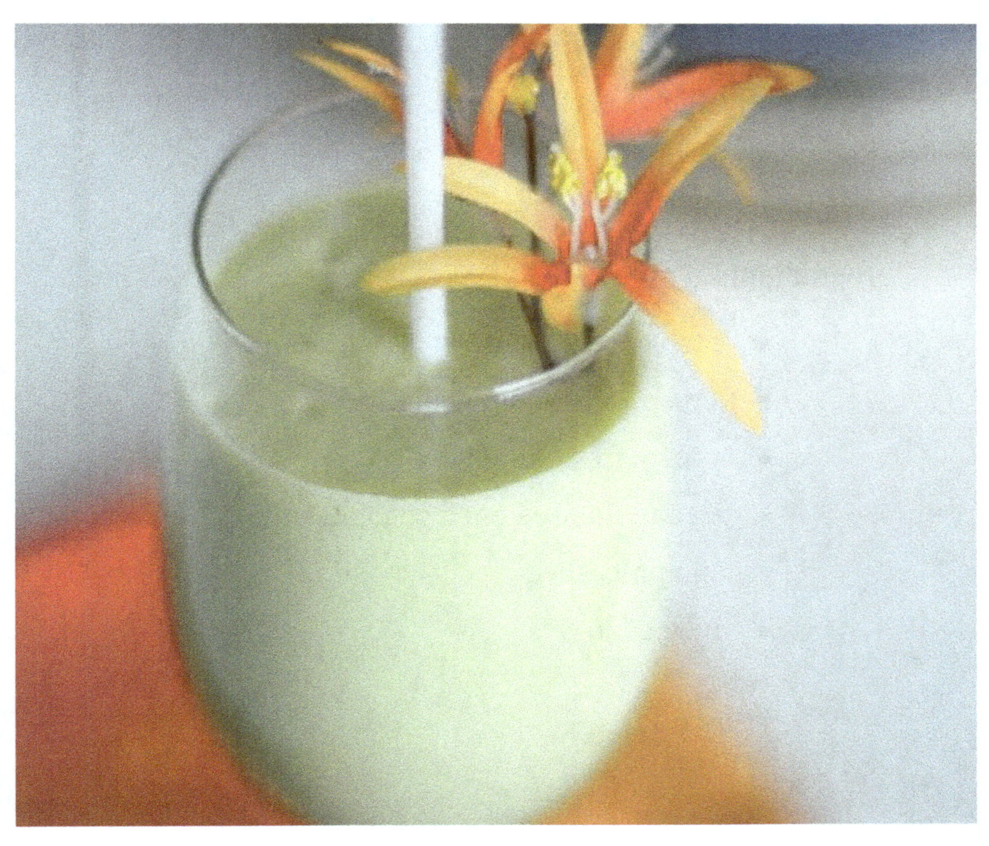

Apple Avocado Coconut Smoothie

Preparation Time: 5 minutes - Cooking Time: 0 minutes - Servings: 2

Ingredients:

- 1 tsp coconut oil
- 1 tbsp. collagen powder
- 1 tbsp. fresh lime juice
- ½ cup unsweetened coconut milk
- ¼ apple, slice
- 1 avocado

Directions:

1. Add all ingredients into the blender and blend until smooth and creamy.
2. Serve and enjoy.

Nutrition: Calories 262 / Fat 23.9 g / Carbohydrates 13.6 g / Sugar 3.4 g / Protein 2 g
Cholesterol 0 mg

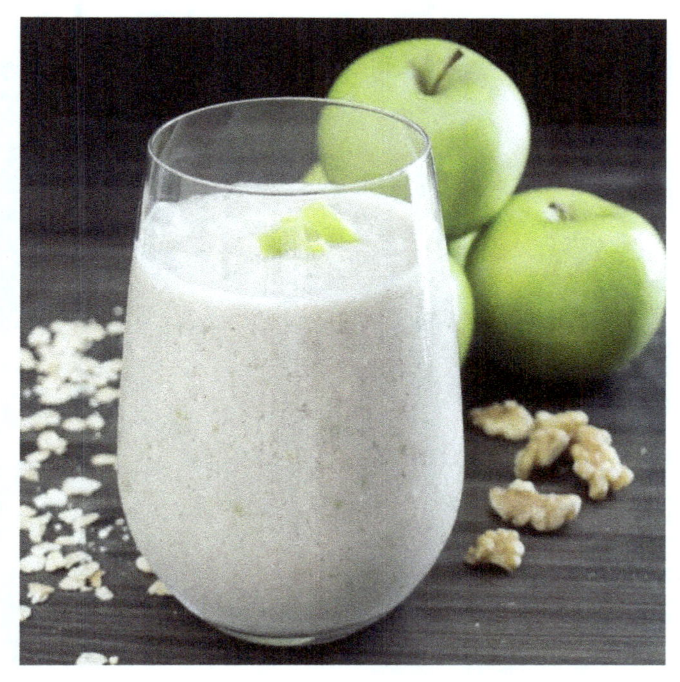

Healthy Spinach Green Smoothie

Preparation Time: 5 minutes - Cooking Time: 0 minutes - Servings: 1

Ingredients:

- 1 cup ice cube
- 2/3 cup water
- ½ cup unsweetened almond milk
- 5 drops liquid stevia
- ½ tsp matcha powder
- 1 tsp vanilla extract
- 1 tbsp. MCT oil
- ½ avocado
- 2/3 cup spinach

Directions:

1. Add all ingredients into the blender and blend until smooth and creamy.
2. Serve immediately and enjoy it.

Nutrition: Calories 167 / Fat 18.3 g / Carbohydrates 3.8 g / Sugar 0.6 g / Protein 1.6 g

Cholesterol 0 mg

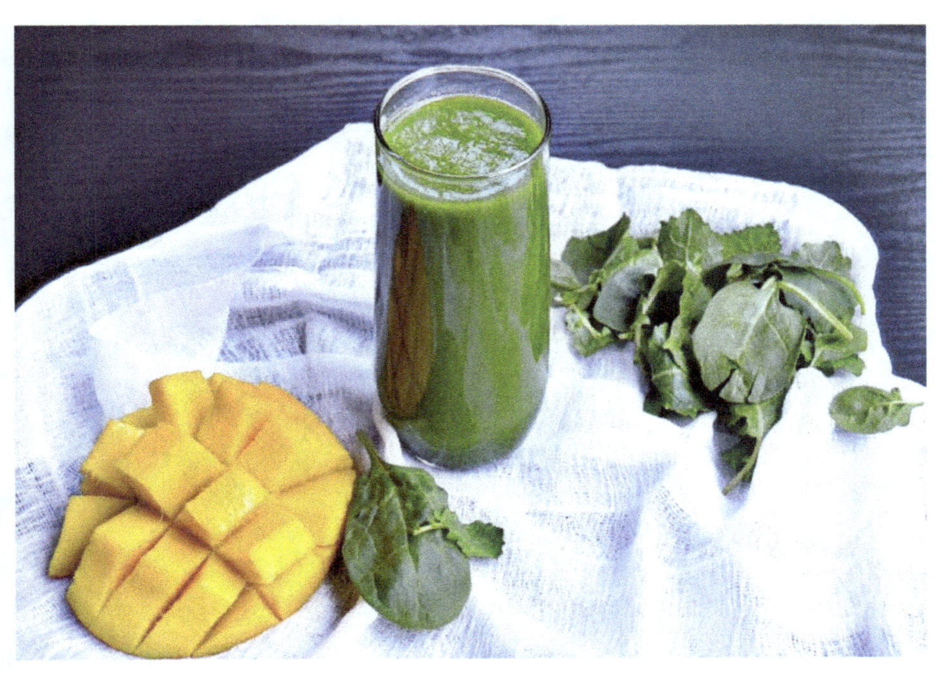

Cinnamon Muffins

Preparation Time: 25 minutes - Cooking Time: 15 minutes
Servings: 20

Ingredients:

- ½ cup coconut oil, melted
- ½ cup pumpkin puree
- ½ cup almond butter
- 1 tbsp. cinnamon
- 1 tsp baking powder
- 2 scoops vanilla protein powder
- ½ cup almond flour

Directions:

1. Preheat the oven to 180 C/ 350 F.
2. Spray a muffin tray with cooking spray and set aside.
3. Add all dry ingredients into the large bowl and mix well.
4. Add wet ingredients and mix until well combined. Pour batter into the prepared muffin tray and bake in preheated oven for 15 minutes.
5. Serve and enjoy.

Nutrition: Calories 80 / Fat 7.1 g / Carbohydrates 1.6 g / Sugar 0.4 g / Protein 3.5 g

Cholesterol 0 mg

Keto Porridge

Preparation Time: 10 minutes - Cooking Time: 5 minutes - Servings: 1

Ingredients:

- ½ tsp vanilla extract
- ¼ tsp granulated stevia
- 1 tbsp. chia seeds
- 1 tbsp. flaxseed meal
- 2 tbsp. unsweetened shredded coconut
- 2 tbsp. almond flour
- 2 tbsp. hemp hearts
- ½ cup of water - Pinch of salt

Directions:

1. Add all ingredients except vanilla extract to a saucepan and heat over low heat until thickened.
2. Stir well and serve warm.

Nutrition: Calories 370 / Fat 30.2 g / Carbohydrates 12.8 g / Sugar 1.9 g / Protein 13.5 g

Cholesterol 0 mg

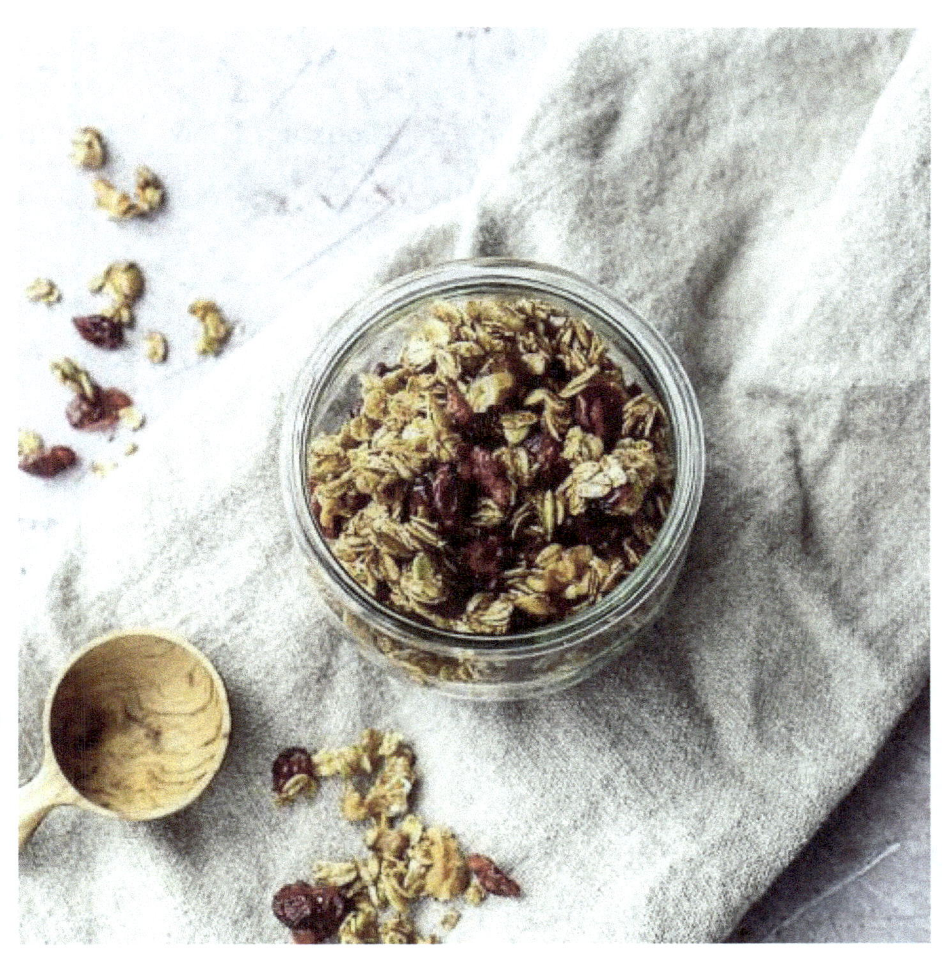

Easy Chia Seed Pudding

Preparation Time: 10 minutes - Cooking Time: 0 minutes - Servings: 4

Ingredients:

- ¼ tsp cinnamon
- 15 drops liquid stevia
- ½ tsp vanilla extract
- ½ cup chia seeds
- 2 cups unsweetened coconut milk

Directions:

1. Add all ingredients into the glass jar and mix well.
2. Close jar with lid and place in the refrigerator for 4 hours.
3. Serve chilled and enjoy.

Nutrition: Calories 347 / Fat 33.2 g / Carbohydrates 9.8 g / Sugar 4.1 g / Protein 5.9 g

Cholesterol 0 mg

Avocado Tofu Scramble

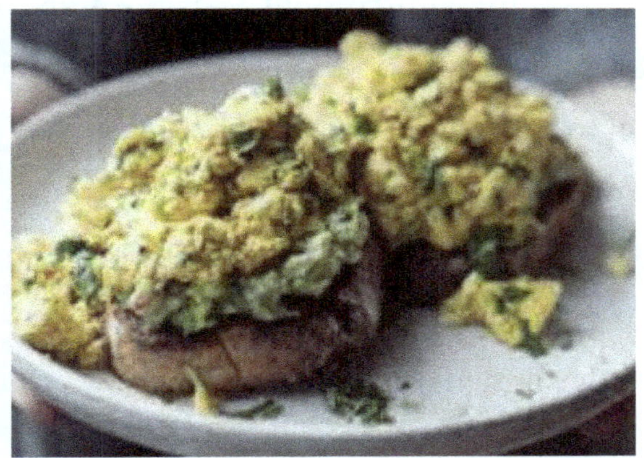

Preparation Time: 15 minutes - Cooking Time: 0 minutes - Servings: 1

Ingredients:

- 1 tbsp. fresh parsley, chopped
- ½ medium avocado
- ½ block firm tofu drained and crumbled
- ½ cup bell pepper, chopped
- ½ cup onion, chopped
- 1 tsp olive oil - 1 tbsp. water
- ¼ tsp cumin - ¼ tsp garlic powder
- ¼ tsp paprika - ¼ tsp turmeric
- 1 tbsp. nutritional yeast
- Pepper - Salt

Directions:

1. In a small bowl, mix nutritional yeast, water, and spices. Set aside.

2. Heat olive oil to the pan over medium heat.

3. Add onion and bell pepper and sauté for 5 minutes.

4. Add crumbled tofu and nutritional yeast to the pan and sauté for 2 minutes.

5. Top with parsley and avocado.

6. Serve and enjoy.

Nutrition: Calories 164 / Fat 9.7 g / Carbohydrates 15 g / Sugar g / Protein 7.4 g

Cholesterol 0 mg

Avo-Tacos

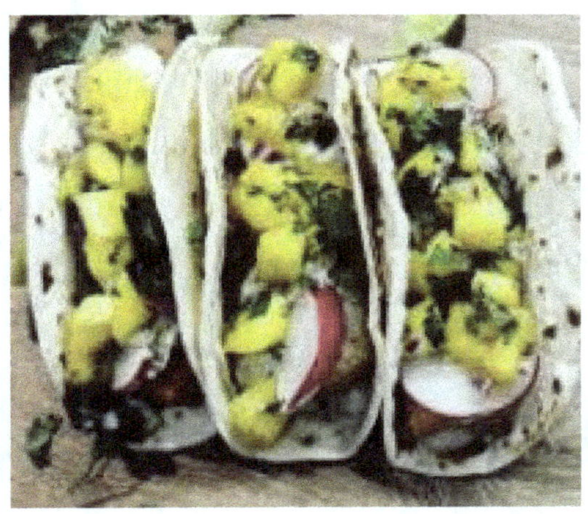

Preparation Time: 15 minutes - Cooking Time: 5 minutes - Servings: 4

Ingredients

- 30 milliliters, Avocado Oil
- 60 grams, Cauliflower Rice
- 58 grams, Walnuts or Pecans, crushed
- 14 grams, Chipotle Chili, chopped
- 14 grams, Jalapeno Pepper, minced
- 20 grams Onions, chopped
- 2.5 grams Cumin
- 2.5 grams Salt, sea salt preferred
- 100 grams, Tomato, ripe and diced
- 15 milliliters, Lime Juice

Directions:

1. The Avo-Taco is so easy to make that you'll want to do this every week. Start by grabbing a bowl and putting the salsa ingredients together; in a small bowl, you'll need the diced tomatoes, jalapeno, the onion and half of the lime. If you want, you can add in a bit of cilantro to give it a bit more freshness, and don't forget to add the salt!

2. Once you're done, put a frying pan on medium heat and add the avocado oil and let it heat. In the meantime, you can get together the rest of the ingredients, including the cauli-rice (which you can totally make at home if you want--it's a 5-minute blend job), and toss in everything but the avocado, and cook on low to medium heat for about 5 minutes. Add the mixture to the avocado halves and top with salsa and munch away!

Nutrition: Calories 179 / Carbohydrates 13 g / Fats 28.24 g / Protein 4 g

Gooseberry Sauce

Preparation Time: 30 min. - Cooking Time: 5 min. - Servings: 4

Ingredients

- 5 cups gooseberries, rinsed, topped and tailed
- 5 garlic cloves, crushed
- 1 cup fresh dill, rinsed, stems removed
- Salt to taste

Directions

1. Combine gooseberries and dill in a blender and pulse until smooth.
2. Add garlic and salt.
3. Let stand for 30 minutes, covered.

Nutrition: Carbs: 8 g / Fat: 2 g / Protein: 1 g / Calories: 35

Nori Salad Dressing

Preparation Time: 5 min. - Cooking Time: 0 min. - Servings: 6

Ingredients

- 2 toasted nori sheets
- 2 Tbsp. sesame oil
- ¾ cup rice wine vinegar
- 1 Tbsp. orange zest
- ½ tsp sea salt

Directions

1. Break the toasted nori into small pieces.
2. Add all ingredients in a blender and pulse on high.
3. Serve the nori dressing over roasted vegetables. Keep refrigerated.

Nutrition: Carbs: 0.5 g / Fat: 1.5 g / Protein: 0.3 g / Calories: 18

Stuffed Peppers

Preparation Time: 15 min. - Cooking Time: 30 min. - Servings: 2

Ingredients

- 1 large bell pepper, halved, deseeded
- 1 medium eggplant, rinsed, cubed
- 1 tomato, peeled, cubed - 1 onion, chopped
- 1 carrot, grated - 2 sprigs basil
- 1 garlic clove, crushed
- Salt and pepper to taste
- 2 Tbsp. olive oil

Directions

1. Add half the onion to a preheated pan with olive oil. Season with salt and pepper.
2. Add eggplant and fry until golden.
3. In a stewpot sauté the remaining onion with carrots. Season with salt and pepper.
4. Add tomatoes and garlic to the carrots. Cook for 10 minutes, covered, over medium heat.
5. Fill the pepper halves with eggplant and onions.
6. Place the stuffed peppers into the stewpot. Stew for 15 minutes until the pepper is soft.

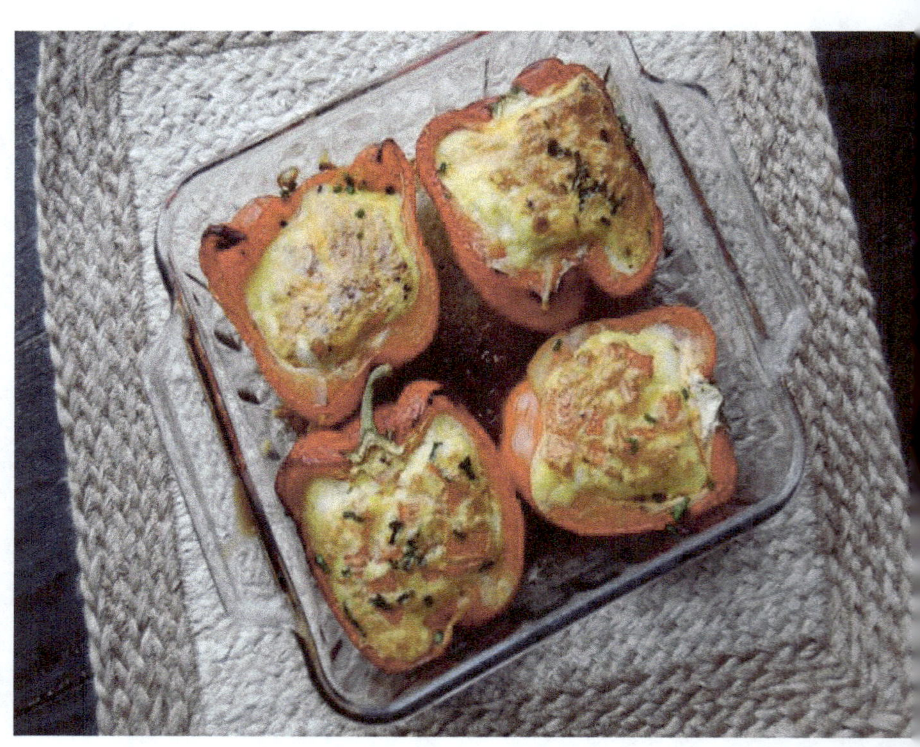

Walnut & Garlic Summer Squash

Preparation Time: 15 min. - Cooking Time: 10 min. - Servings: 4

Ingredients

- 2 lbs. green summer squash, rinsed, cubed
- ½ cup walnuts, crushed
- 3 garlic cloves, crushed
- 10 sprigs parsley, minced
- 2 Tbsp. + 1 Tbsp. vegetable oil

Directions

1. In a preheated pan with oil, add cubed squash and cook over high heat until soft.
2. In a bowl, combine minced parsley, garlic, walnuts and 1 Tbsp. oil. Mix well.
3. Add the walnut mixture to the pan and mix well. Turn the heat off.
4. Serve warm or cooled to your liking.

Nutrition: Carbs: 10 g / Fat: 20 g / Protein: 5.3 g / Calories: 239

Onion Fritters

Preparation Time: 5 min. - Cooking Time: 20 min. - Servings: 4

Ingredients

- 3 large onions, peeled
- 4 leeks
- 6 Tbsp. Keto friendly flour (almond/coconut)
- ¼ tsp fish seasoning
- Salt and pepper to taste

Directions

1. Chop the onions and leeks and add to the food processor. Pulse until smooth.
2. To the pureed onions add flour and seasonings.
3. In a preheated pan with oil, spoon out the fritters and fry until golden on each side over high heat.

Nutrition: Carbs: 13 g / Fat: 11 g / Protein: 5 g / Calories: 186

Fried Tofu

Preparation Time: 5 min. - Cooking Time: 10 min. - Servings: 4

Ingredients

- 1 lb. tofu, cubed - 2 tomatoes, chopped
- 1 chili pepper, chopped - ½ cup onion, chopped
- 2 garlic cloves, minced - 1 Tbsp. olive oil
- 1 Tbsp. lime juice - 1 tsp ground chili
- ½ tsp cumin - ½ tsp oregano - Salt to taste

Directions

1. In a preheated pan with olive oil pan add fresh chili pepper, onions, garlic and fry stirring for 4 minutes.
2. Season with ground chili, cumin, oregano, and salt. Cook, stirring, 30 seconds.
3. Add tofu to the pan and lower the heat. Cook, stirring, for 5 minutes.
4. Right before serving, top with lime juice.
5. Serve with fresh tomatoes.

Nutrition: Carbs: 2.5 g / Fat: 5.7 g / Protein: 5 g / Calories: 76

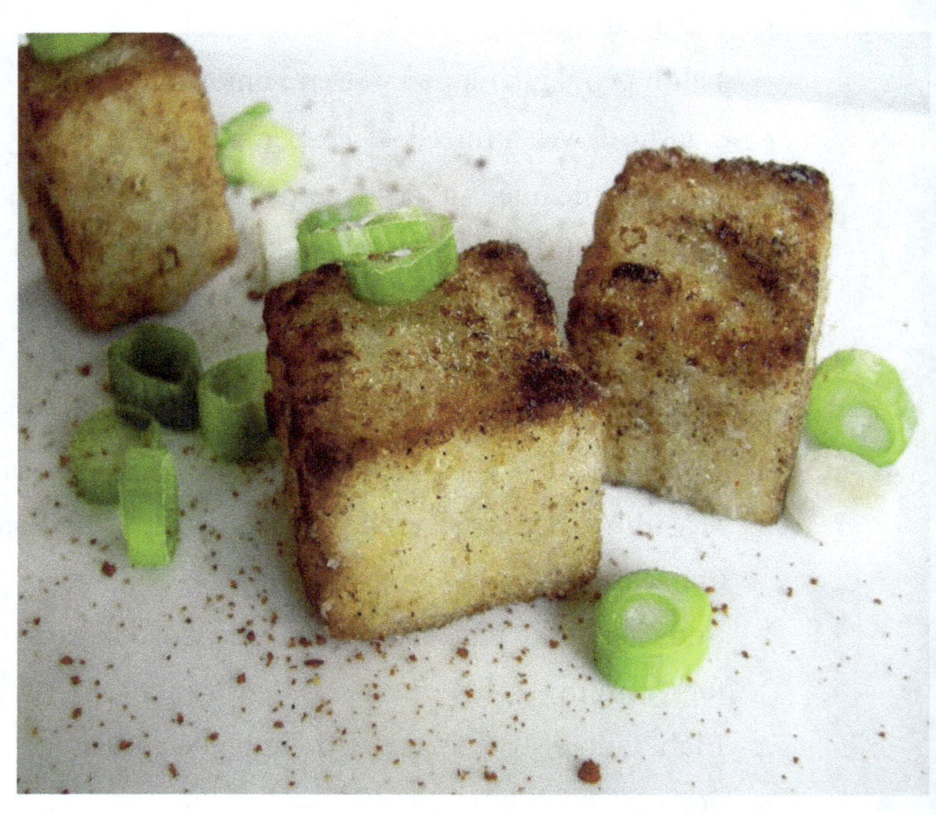

Coconut Leek Soup

Preparation Time: 5 min. - Cooking Time: 30 min. - Servings: 4

Ingredients

- 1 leek, circled - 1 carrot, sliced
- 3 celery stalks, sliced - ½ lemon, juiced
- 1½ cup coconut milk - 1 tsp curry
- 3 Tbsp. grated ginger root - ½ tsp salt
- 2 Tbsp. olive oil - 2 cups water

Directions

1. Add the leeks, carrots, and celery to a pot with olive oil and some water. Let stew until the vegetables are soft.
2. Add 1½ cup water and 1½ cup coconut milk and bring to boil. Cook for 2 minutes on low.
3. Add lemon juice, ginger, curry, and salt and cook on low for 2 minutes.

Nutrition: Carbs: 11 g / Fat: 9.6 g / Protein: 3.6 g / Calories: 142

Seitan Tex-Mex Casserole

Preparation Time: 5 minutes - Cooking Time: 35 minutes

Servings: 4

Ingredients:

- 2 tbsp. vegan butter - 1 ½ lb. seitan
- 3 tbsp. Tex-Mex seasoning
- 2 tbsp. chopped jalapeño peppers
- ½ cup crushed tomatoes
- Salt and black pepper to taste
- ½ cup shredded vegan cheese
- 1 tbsp. chopped fresh green onion to garnish
- 1 cup sour cream for serving

Directions:

1. Preheat the oven and grease a baking dish with cooking spray. Set aside.
2. Melt the vegan butter in a medium skillet over medium heat and cook the seitan until brown, 10 minutes.
3. Stir in the Tex-Mex seasoning, jalapeño peppers, and tomatoes; simmer for 5 minutes and adjust the taste with salt and black pepper.

4. Transfer and level the mixture in the baking dish. Top with the vegan cheese and bake in the upper rack of the oven for 15 to 20 minutes or until the cheese melts and is golden brown.

5. Remove the dish and garnish with the green onion.

6. Serve the casserole with sour cream.

Nutrition: Calories: 464 / Total Fat: 37.8 g, / Saturated Fat: 7.4 g, / Total Carbs: 12 g,

Dietary Fiber: 2g / Sugar: 3g / Protein: 24 g, / Sodium: 147mg

Avocado Coconut Pie

Preparation Time: 30 minutes - Cooking Time: 50 minutes - Servings: 4

Ingredients:

For the piecrust:

- 1 tbsp. flax seed powder + 3 tbsp. water
- 4 tbsp. coconut flour
- 4 tbsp. chia seeds
- ¾ cup almond flour
- 1 tbsp. psyllium husk powder
- 1 tsp baking powder
- 1 pinch salt
- 3 tbsp. coconut oil
- 4 tbsp. water

For the filling:

- 2 ripe avocados - 1 cup vegan mayonnaise
- 3 tbsp. flax seed powder + 9 tbsp. water
- 2 tbsp. fresh parsley, finely chopped
- 1 jalapeno, finely chopped
- ½ tsp onion powder - ¼ tsp salt
- ½ cup cashew cream
- 1¼ cups shredded tofu cheese

Directions:

1. In 2 separate bowls, mix the different portions of flax seed powder with the respective quantity of water. Allow absorbing for 5 minutes.

2. Preheat the oven to 350 F.

3. In a food processor, add the coconut flour, chia seeds, almond flour, psyllium husk powder, baking powder, salt, coconut oil, water, and the smaller portion of the flax egg. Blend the ingredients until the resulting dough forms into a ball.

4. Line a spring form pan with about 12-inch diameter of parchment paper and spread the dough in the pan. Bake for 10 to 15 minutes or until a light golden brown color is achieved.

5. Meanwhile, cut the avocado into halves lengthwise, remove the pit, and chop the pulp. Put in a bowl and add the mayonnaise, remaining flax egg, parsley, jalapeno, onion powder, salt, cashew cream, and tofu cheese. Combine well.

6. Remove the piecrust when ready and fill with the creamy mixture. Level the filling with a spatula and continue baking for 35 minutes or until lightly golden brown.

7. When ready, take out. Cool before slicing and serving with a baby spinach salad.

Nutrition: Calories: 680 / Total Fat: 71.8 g / Saturated Fat: 20.9 g / Total Carbs: 10g

Dietary Fiber: 7 g / Sugar: 2g / Protein: 3g / Sodium: 525 mg

Baked Mushrooms with Creamy Brussels sprouts

Preparation Time: 8 minutes - Cooking Time: 2 hours 35 minutes - Servings: 4

Ingredients:

For the mushrooms:

- 1 lb. whole white button mushrooms
- Salt and black pepper to taste - 2 tsp dried thyme - 1 bay leaf
- 5 black peppercorns - ½ cups vegetable broth
- 2 garlic cloves, minced - 1 ½ oz. fresh ginger, grated
- 1 tbsp. coconut oil - 1 tbsp. smoked paprika

For the creamy Brussel sprouts:

- ½ lb. Brussel sprouts, halved
- 1 ½ cups cashew cream
- Salt and ground black pepper to taste

Directions:

For the mushroom roast:

1. Preheat the oven to 200 F.
2. Pour all the mushroom ingredients into a baking dish, stir well, and cover with foil. Bake in the oven until softened, 1 to 2 hours.

3. Remove the dish, take off the foil, and use a slotted
    spoon to fetch the mushrooms onto serving plates. Set
    aside.

For the creamy Brussel sprouts:

4. Pour the broth in the baking dish into a medium pot
    and add the Brussel sprouts. Add about ½ cup of
    water if needed and cook for 7 to 10 minutes or until
    softened.

5. Stir in the cashew cream, adjust the taste with salt and
    black pepper, and simmer for 15 min

6. Serve the creamy Brussel sprouts with the
    mushrooms.

Nutrition: Calories: 492 / Total Fat: 37.9g / Saturated Fat: 9.1g /
Total Carbs: 13g

Dietary Fiber: 2 / Sugar: 2 g / Protein: 29g / Sodium: 779mg

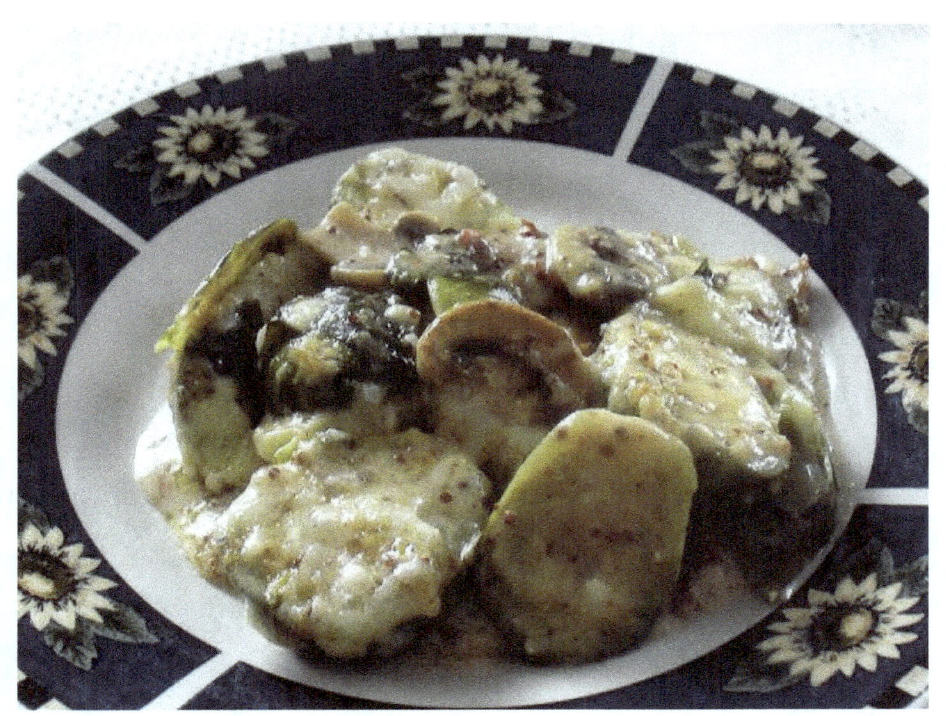

Pimiento Tofu balls

Preparation Time: 10 minutes - Cooking Time: 15 minutes - Servings: 4

Ingredients:

- ¼ cup chopped pimientos - 1/3 cup mayonnaise
- 3 tbsp. cashew cream - 1 tsp paprika powder
- 1 pinch cayenne pepper - 1 tbsp. Dijon mustard
- 4 oz. grated vegan cheese - 1 ½ lbs. tofu, pressed and crumbled
- Salt and black pepper to taste - 2 tbsp. olive oil, for frying

Directions:

1. In a large bowl, add all the ingredients except for the olive oil and with gloves on your hands, mix the ingredients until well combined. Form bite size balls from the mixture.
2. Heat the olive oil in a medium non-stick skillet and fry the tofu balls in batches on both sides until brown and cooked through, 4 to 5 minutes on each side.
3. Transfer the tofu balls to a serving plate and serve warm.

Nutrition: Calories: 254 / Total Fat: 36.8g / Saturated Fat: 8.7g / Total Carbs: 12g,

Dietary Fiber: 1g / Sugar: 1g / Protein: 26 g / Sodium: 773 mg

Tempeh with Garlic Asparagus

Preparation Time: 10 minutes - Cooking Time: 18 minutes - Servings: 4

Ingredients:

For the tempeh:

- 3 tbsp. vegan butter - 4 tempeh slices
- Salt and black pepper to taste

For the garlic buttered asparagus:

- 2 tbsp. olive oil - 2 garlic cloves, minced
- 1 lb. asparagus, trimmed and halved
- Salt and black pepper to taste
- 1 tbsp. dried parsley - 1 small lemon, juiced

Directions:

For the tempeh:

1. Melt the vegan butter in a medium skillet over medium heat, season the tempeh with salt, black pepper and fry in the butter on both sides until brown and cooked through, 10 minutes. Transfer to a plate and set aside in a warmer for serving.

For the garlic asparagus:

2. Heat the olive oil in a medium skillet over medium heat, and sauté the garlic until fragrant, 30 seconds.
3. Stir in the asparagus, season with salt and black pepper, and cook until slightly softened with a bit of crunch, 5 minutes.
4. Mix in the parsley, lemon juice, toss to coat well, and plate the asparagus.
5. Serve the asparagus warm with the tempeh.

Nutrition: Calories: 181 / Total Fat: 17.5 g / Saturated Fat: 11 g / Total Carbs: 6 g,
Dietary Fiber: 3g / Sugar: 2g / Protein: 3g / Sodium: 140mg

Mushroom Curry Pie

Preparation Time: 15 minutes - Cooking Time: 55 minutes

Servings: 4

Ingredients:

For the piecrust:

- 1 tbsp. flax seed powder + 3 tbsp. water
- ¾ cup coconut flour
- 4 tbsp. chia seeds
- 4 tbsp. almond flour
- 1 tbsp. psyllium husk powder
- 1 tsp baking powder
- 1 pinch salt
- 3 tbsp. olive oil
- 4 tbsp. water

For the filling:

- 1 cup chopped cremini mushrooms
- 1 cup vegan mayonnaise
- 3 tbsp. + 9 tbsp. water
- ½ red bell pepper, finely chopped
- 1 tsp turmeric powder
- ½ tsp paprika powder
- ½ tsp garlic powder

- ¼ tsp black pepper
- ½ cup cashew cream
- 1¼ cups shredded tofu cheese

Directions:

1. In two separate bowls, mix the different portions of flax seed powder with the respective quantity of water and set aside to absorb for 5 minutes.
2. Preheat the oven to 350 F.
3. Make the crust:
4. When the flax egg is ready, pour the smaller quantity into a food processor, and add the coconut flour, chia seeds, almond flour, psyllium husk powder, baking powder, salt, olive oil, and water. Blend the ingredients until a ball forms out of the dough.
5. Line a springform pan with an 8-inch diameter parchment paper and grease the pan with cooking spray.
6. Spread the dough in the bottom of the pan and bake in the oven for 15 minutes.
7. Make the filling:
8. In a bowl, add the remaining flax egg, mushrooms, mayonnaise, water, bell pepper, turmeric, paprika, garlic powder, black pepper, cashew cream, and tofu

cheese. Combine the mixture evenly and fill the piecrust. Bake further for 40 minutes or until the pie is golden brown.

9. Remove, slice, and serve the pie with a chilled strawberry drink.

Nutrition: Calories: 548/ Total Fat: 55.9g / Saturated Fat: 8.5 g / Total Carbs: 6g

Dietary Fiber: 2 g / Sugar: 2g / Protein: 8 g / Sodium: 405mg

Spicy Cheese with Tofu Balls

 Preparation Time: 20 minutes - Cooking Time: 20 minutes - Servings: 4

Ingredients:

For the spicy cheese:

- 1/3 cup vegan mayonnaise
- ¼ cup pickled jalapenos
- 1 tsp paprika powder
- 1 tbsp. mustard powder
- 1 pinch cayenne pepper
- 4 oz. grated tofu cheese

For the tofu balls:

- 1 tbsp. flax seed powder + 3 tbsp. water
- 2 ½ cup crumbled tofu
- Salt and black pepper
- 2 tbsp. plant butter, for frying

Directions:

1. Make the spicy cheese. In a bowl, mix the mayonnaise, jalapenos, paprika, mustard powder, cayenne powder, and cheddar cheese. Set aside.

2. In another medium bowl, combine the flax seed powder with water and allow absorbing for 5 minutes.

3. Add the flax egg to the cheese mixture, the crumbled tofu, salt, and black pepper, and combine well. Use your hands to form large meatballs out of the mix.

4. Then, melt the vegan butter in a large skillet over medium heat and fry the tofu balls until cooked and browned on the outside.

5. Serve the tofu balls with roasted cauliflower mash and mayonnaise.

Nutrition: Calories: 259 / Total Fat: 55.9g / Saturated Fat: 11.4 g / Total Carbs: 5 g,
Dietary Fiber: 1g / Sugar: 1g / Protein: 16g / Sodium: 452mg

Tempeh Coconut Curry Bake

Preparation Time: 7minutes - Cooking Time: 23minutes - Servings: 4

Ingredients:

- 1 oz. plant butter, for greasing
- 2 ½ cups chopped tempeh
- Salt and black pepper
- 4 tbsp. plant butter
- 2 tbsp. red curry paste
- 1 ½ cup coconut cream
- ½ cup fresh parsley, chopped
- 15 oz. cauliflower, cut into florets

Directions:

1. Preheat the oven to 400 F and grease a baking dish with 1 ounce of vegan butter.
2. Arrange the tempeh in the baking dish, sprinkle with salt and black pepper, and top each tempeh with a slice of the remaining butter.
3. In a bowl, mix the red curry paste with the coconut cream and parsley. Pour the mixture over the tempeh.

4. Bake in the oven for 20 minutes or until the tempeh is
    cooked.

5. While baking, season the cauliflower with salt, place in
    a microwave-safe bowl, and sprinkle with some water.
    Steam in the microwave for 3 minutes or until the
    cauliflower is soft and tender within.

6. Remove the curry bake and serve with the caulis.

Nutrition: Calories: 417 / Total Fat: 38.8g / Saturated Fat: 22.4g
/ Total Carbs: 11g
Dietary Fiber: 2g / Sugar: 3g / Protein: 11g / Sodium: 194mg

Kale and Mushroom Pierogis

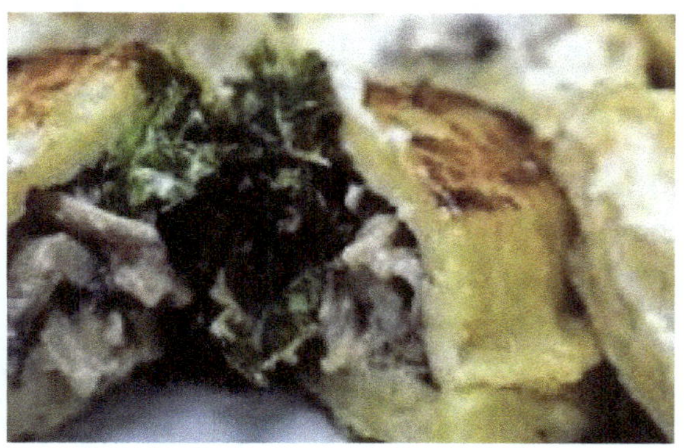

Preparation Time: 15 minutes - Cooking Time: 30 minutes - Servings: 4

Ingredients:

For the stuffing:

- 2 tbsp. vegan butter
- 2 garlic cloves, finely chopped
- 1 small red onion, finely chopped
- 3 oz. baby bella mushrooms, sliced
- 2 oz. fresh kale
- ½ tsp salt
- ¼ tsp black pepper
- ½ cup cashew cream
- 2 oz. grated tofu cheese

For the pierogi:

- 1 tbsp. flax seed powder + 3 tbsp. water
- ½ cup almond flour
- 4 tbsp. coconut flour
- ½ tsp salt
- 1 tsp baking powder
- 1½ cups shredded tofu cheese
- 5 tbsp. vegan butter
- Olive oil for brushing

Directions:

1. Put the vegan butter in a skillet and melt over medium heat, then add and sauté the garlic, red onion, mushrooms, and kale until the mushrooms brown.
2. Season the mixture with salt and black pepper and reduce the heat to low. Stir in the cashew cream and tofu cheese and simmer for 1 minute. Turn the heat off and set the filling aside to cool.
3. Make the pierogis: In a small bowl, mix the flax seed powder with water and allow sitting for 5 minutes.
4. In a bowl, combine the almond flour, coconut flour, salt, and baking powder.

5. Put a small pan over low heat, add, and melt the tofu cheese and vegan butter while stirring continuously until smooth batter forms. Turn the heat off.

6. Pour the flax egg into the cream mixture, continue stirring, while adding the flour mixture until a firm dough forms.

7. Mold the dough into four balls, place on a chopping board, and use a rolling pin to flatten each into ½ inch thin round pieces.

8. Spread a generous amount of stuffing on one-half of each dough, then fold over the filling, and seal the dough with your fingers.

9. Brush with olive oil, place on a baking sheet, and bake for 20 minutes or until the pierogis turn a golden brown color.

10. Serve the pierogis with a lettuce tomato salad.

Nutrition: Calories: 364 / Total Fat: 33.4 g / Saturated Fat: 17.3 g / Total Carbs: 8g

Dietary Fiber: 2g / Sugar: 3 g / Protein: 12 g / Sodium: 779 mg

Mushroom Lettuce Wraps

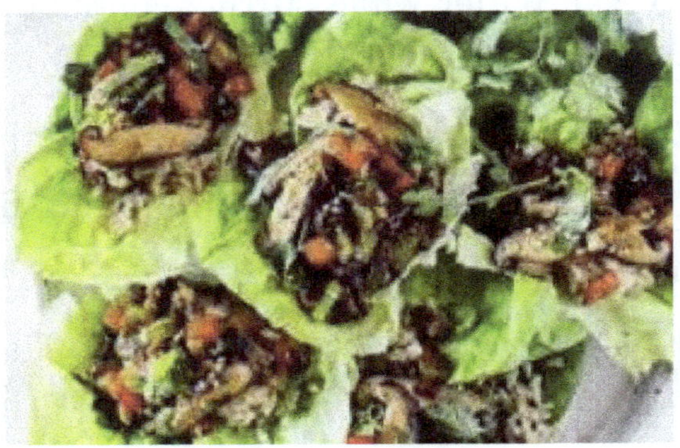

Preparation Time: 5minutes - Cooking Time: 16minutes - Servings: 4

Ingredients:

- 2 tbsp. vegan butter
- 4 oz. baby bella mushrooms, sliced
- 1½ lbs. tofu, crumbled
- ½ tsp salt
- ¼ tsp black pepper
- 1 iceberg lettuce, leaves extracted
- 1 cup shredded vegan cheese
- 1 large tomato, sliced

Directions:

1. Put the vegan butter in a skillet and melt over medium heat. Add the mushrooms and sauté until browned and tender, about 6 minutes. Transfer the mushrooms to a plate and set aside.
2. Add the tofu to the skillet, season with salt and black pepper, and cook until brown, about 10 minutes. Turn the heat off.
3. Spoon the tofu and mushrooms into the lettuce leaves, sprinkle with the vegan cheese, and share the tomato slices on top.
4. Serve the burger immediately.

Nutrition: Calories: 439 / Total Fat: 31.9 g / Saturated Fat: 12.2 g / Total Carbs: 9 g

Dietary Fiber: 4g / Sugar: 1 g / Protein: 36g / Sodium: 574mg

Tofu and Spinach Lasagna with Red Sauce

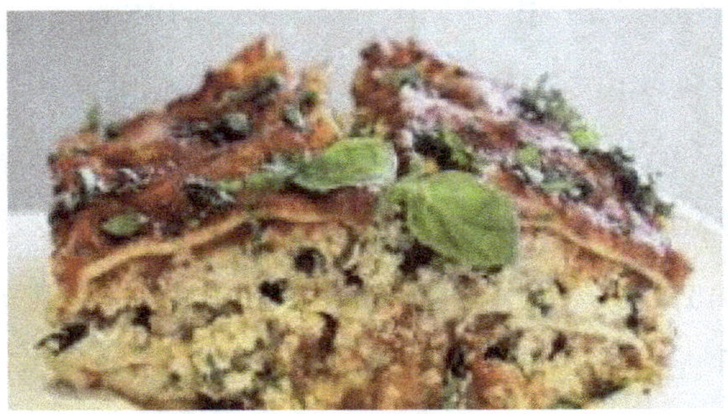

Preparation Time: 20 minutes - Cooking Time: 45 minutes - Servings: 4

Ingredients:

- 2 tbsp. vegan butter
- 1 white onion, chopped
- 1 garlic clove, minced
- 2 ½ cups crumbled tofu
- 3 tbsp. tomato paste
- ½ tbsp. dried oregano
- 1 tsp salt
- ¼ tsp ground black pepper
- ½ cup water
- 1 cup baby spinach

Keto pasta

- Flax egg: 8 tbsp. flax seed powder + 1 ½ cups water
- 1 ½ cup dairy-free cashew cream
- 1 tsp salt
- 5 tbsp. psyllium husk powder

Dairy-free cheese topping

- 2 cups coconut cream
- 5 oz. shredded vegan mozzarella cheese
- 2 oz. grated tofu cheese
- ½ tsp salt
- ¼ tsp ground black pepper
- ½ cup fresh parsley, finely chopped

Directions:

1. Melt the vegan butter in a medium pot over medium heat. Then, add the white onion and garlic, and sauté until fragrant and soft, about 3 minutes.
2. Stir in the tofu and cook until brown. Mix in the tomato paste, oregano, salt, and black pepper.
3. Pour the water into the pot, stir, and simmer the ingredients until most of the liquid has evaporated.
4. While cooking the sauce, make the lasagna sheets. Preheat the oven to 300 F and mix the flax seed

powder with the water in a medium bowl to make flax egg. Allow sitting to thicken for 5 minutes.

5. Combine the flax egg with the cashew cream and salt. Add the psyllium husk powder a bit at a time while whisking and allow the mixture to sit for a few more minutes.

6. Line a baking sheet with parchment paper and spread the mixture in. Cover with another parchment paper and use a rolling pin to flatten the dough into the sheet.

7. Bake the batter in the oven for 10 to 12 minutes, remove after, take off the parchment papers, and slice the pasta into sheets that fit your baking dish.

8. In a bowl, combine the coconut cream and two-thirds of the mozzarella cheese. Fetch out 2 tablespoons of the mixture and reserve.

9. Mix in the tofu cheese, salt, black pepper, and parsley. Set aside.

10. Grease your baking dish with cooking spray, layer a single line of pasta in the dish, spread with some tomato sauce, 1/3 of the spinach, and ¼ of the coconut cream mixture. Season with salt and black pepper as desired.

11. Repeat layering the ingredients twice in the same manner making sure to top the final layer with the

coconut cream mixture and the reserved cashew cream.

12. Bake in the oven for 30 minutes at 400 F or until the lasagna has a beautiful brown surface.

13. Remove the dish; allow cooling for a few minutes, and slice.

14. Serve the lasagna with a baby green salad.

Nutrition: Calories: 767 / Total Fat: 69.8 g / Saturated Fat: 34.5 g / Total Carbs: 14g

Dietary Fiber: 3g / Sugar: 5g / Protein: 28 g / Sodium: 1205 mg

Green Avocado Carbonara

Preparation Time: 15minutes - Cooking Time: 15minutes - Servings: 4

Ingredients:

- 8 tbsp. flax seed powder + 1 ½ cups water
- 1 ½ cups dairy-free cashew cream
- 1 tsp salt
- 5 ½ tbsp. psyllium husk powder

Avocado sauce

- 1 avocado, peeled and pitted
- 1 ¾ cups coconut cream
- Juice of ½ lemon
- 1 teaspoon onion powder
- ½ teaspoon garlic powder
- ¼ cup olive oil
- ¾ teaspoon sea salt
- ¼ teaspoon black pepper
- Walnut Parmesan or store-bought parmesan

For serving

- 4 tbsp. toasted pecans
- ½ cup freshly grated tofu cheese

Directions:

1. Preheat the oven to 300 F.
2. In a medium bowl, mix the flax seed powder with water and allow sitting to thicken for 5 minutes.
3. Add the cashew cream, salt, and psyllium husk powder. Whisk until smooth batter forms.
4. Line a baking sheet with parchment paper, pour in the batter and cover with another parchment paper. Use a rolling pin to flatten the dough into the sheet.
5. Place in the oven and bake for 10 to 12 minutes. Remove the pasta after, take off the parchment papers and use a sharp knife to slice the pasta into thin strips lengthwise. Cut each piece into halves, pour into a bowl, and set aside.
6. For the avocado sauce, in a blender, combine the avocado, coconut cream, lemon juice, onion powder, and garlic powder. Puree the ingredients until smooth.
7. Pour the olive oil over the pasta and stir to coat properly. Pour the avocado sauce on top and mix. Then, season with salt, black pepper, and the soy cheese. Combine again.
8. Divide the pasta into serving plates, garnish with extra soy cheese and pecans, and serve immediately.

Nutrition: Calories: 941 / Total Fat: 94.2g / Saturated Fat: 30.4g / Total Carbs: 19g

Dietary Fiber: 8g / Sugar: 5g / Protein: 16g / Sodium: 1314mg

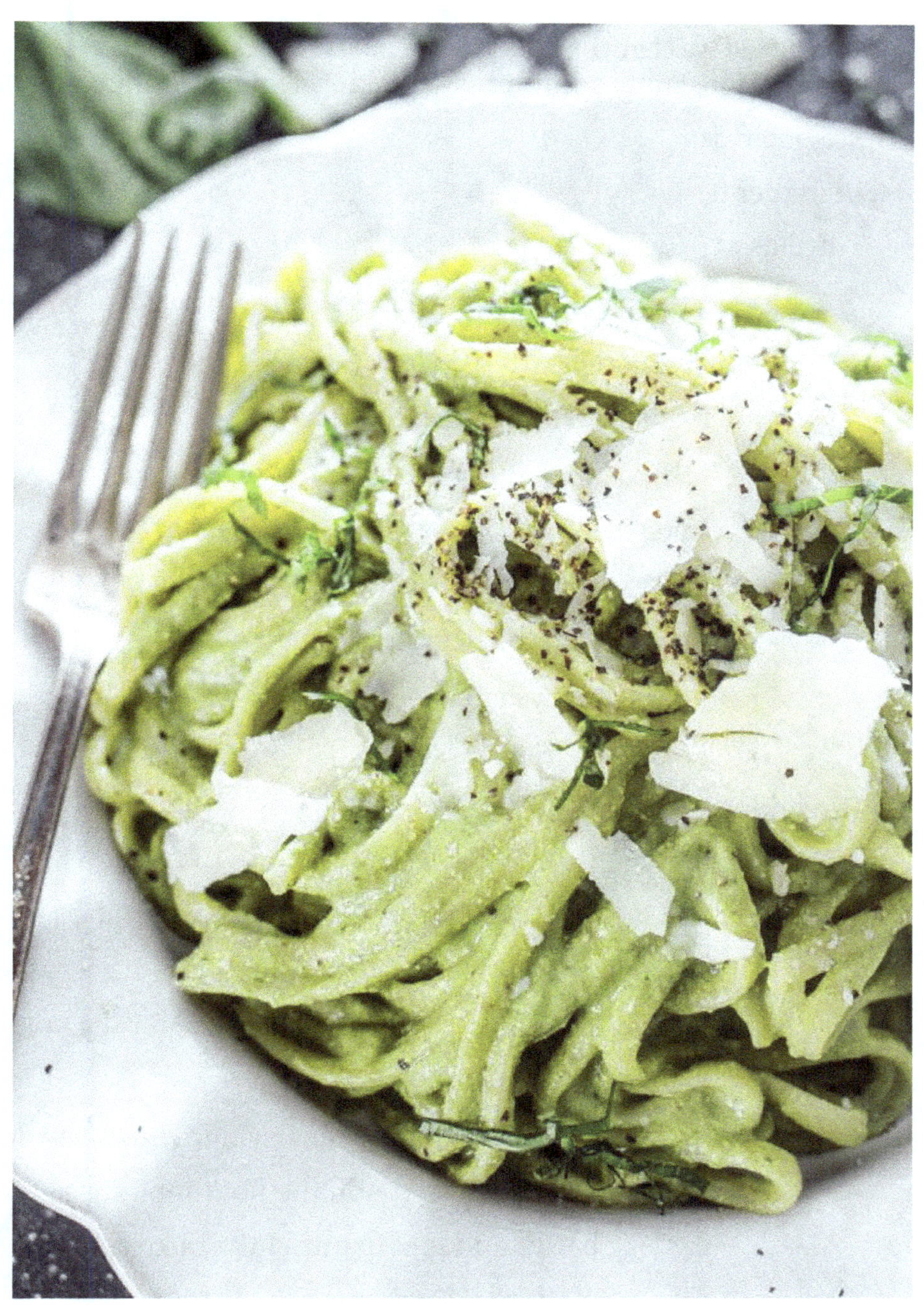

Cashew Buttered Quesadillas with Leafy Greens
Preparation Time: 10minutes - Cooking Time: 20minutes -

Servings: 4

Ingredients:

Tortillas

- 3 tbsp. flax seed powder + ½ cup water
- ½ cup dairy-free cashew cream
- 1½ tsp psyllium husk powder
- 1 tbsp. coconut flour
- ½ tsp salt

Filling

- 1 tbsp. cashew butter, for frying
- 5 oz. grated vegan cheese
- 1 oz. leafy greens

Directions:

1. Preheat the oven to 400 F.
2. In a bowl, mix the flax seed powder with water and allow sitting to thicken for 5 minutes.
3. After, whisk the cashew cream into the flax egg until the batter is smooth.
4. In another bowl, combine the psyllium husk powder, coconut flour, and salt. Add the flour mixture to the flax egg batter and fold in until fully incorporated. Allow sitting for a few minutes.

5. Then, line a baking sheet with parchment paper and pour in the mixture. Spread into the baking sheet using a spatula and bake in the upper rack of the oven for 5 to 7 minutes or until brown around the edges. Keep a watchful eye on the tortillas to prevent burning.

6. Remove when ready and slice into 8 pieces. Set aside.

7. For the filling, spoon a little cashew butter into a skillet and place a tortilla in the pan. Sprinkle with some vegan cheese, leafy greens, and cover with another tortilla.

8. Brown each side of the quesadilla for 1 minute or until the cheese melts. Transfer to a plate.

9. Repeat assembling the quesadillas using the remaining cashew butter.

10. Serve immediately with avocado salad.

Nutrition: Calories: 224 / Total Fat: 20.4g / Saturated Fat: 12.2g / Total Carbs: 1g

Dietary Fiber: 0g / Sugar: 1g / Protein: 9g / Sodium: 556mg

Zucchini Boats with Vegan Cheese

Preparation Time: 3minutes - Cooking Time: 4minutes - Servings: 2

Ingredients:

- 1 medium-sized zucchini - 4 tbsp. vegan butter
- 2 garlic cloves, minced - 1½ oz. baby kale
- Salt and black pepper to taste - 2 tbsp. unsweetened tomato sauce
- 1 cup vegan cheese - Olive oil for drizzling

Directions:

1. Preheat the oven to 375 F.
2. Use a knife to slice the zucchini in halves and scoop out the pulp with a spoon into a plate. Keep the flesh.
3. Grease a baking sheet with cooking spray and place the zucchini boats on top.
4. Put the vegan butter in a skillet and melt over medium heat. Add and sauté the garlic until fragrant and slightly browned, about 4 minutes.
5. Add the kale and the zucchini pulp. Cook until the kale wilts; season with salt and black pepper.
6. Spoon the tomato sauce into the boats and spread to coat the bottom evenly. Then, spoon the kale mixture into the zucchinis and sprinkle with the cheese.
7. Bake in the oven for 20 to 25 minutes or until the cheese has a beautiful golden color.

8. Plate the zucchinis when ready, drizzle with olive oil, and season with salt and black pepper.

9. Serve immediately.

Nutrition: Calories: 721 / Total Fat: 76.8g / Saturated Fat: 21.2g / Total Carbs: 2g

Dietary Fiber: 0g / Sugar: 0g / Protein: 9g / Sodium: 309mg

Tempeh Garam Masala Bake
Preparation Time: 5minutes - Cooking Time: 24minutes -
Servings: 4
Ingredients:

- 3 tbsp. vegan butter - 3 cups tempeh slices
- Salt - 2 tbsp. garam masala
- 1 green bell pepper, finely diced
- 1¼ cups coconut cream
- 1 tbsp. fresh cilantro, finely chopped

Directions:

1. Preheat the oven to 400 F.
2. Place a skillet over medium heat, add, and melt the vegan butter. Meanwhile, season the tempeh with some salt. Fry the tempeh in the butter until browned on both sides, about 4 minutes.
3. Stir half of the garam masala into the tempeh until evenly mixed; turn the heat off.
4. Transfer the tempeh with the spice into a baking dish.
5. Then, in a small bowl, mix the green bell pepper, coconut cream, cilantro, and remaining garam masala.
6. Pour the mixture over the tempeh and bake in the oven for 20 minutes or until golden brown on top.
7. Garnish with cilantro and serve with some cauli rice.

Nutrition: Calories: 286 / Total Fat: 27g / Saturated Fat: 15g / Total Carbs: 5g

Dietary Fiber: 0g / Sugar: 1g / Protein: 9g / Sodium: 87mg

Caprese Casserole

Preparation Time: 5minutes - Cooking Time: 20minutes -

Servings: 4

Ingredients:

- 1 cup cherry tomatoes, halved
- 1 cup vegan mozzarella cheese, cut into small pieces
- 2 tbsp. basil pesto - 1 cup vegan mayonnaise
- 2 oz. tofu cheese - Salt and black pepper
- 1 cup arugula - 4 tbsp. olive oil

Directions:

1. Preheat the oven to 350 F.
2. In a baking dish, mix the cherry tomatoes, mozzarella, basil pesto, and mayonnaise, half of the tofu cheese, salt, and black pepper.
3. Level the ingredients with a spatula and sprinkle the remaining tofu cheese on top. Bake for 20 minutes or until the top of the casserole is golden brown.
4. Remove and allow cooling for a few minutes. Slice and dish into plates, top with some arugula and drizzle with olive oil. Serve.

Nutrition: Calories: 588 / Total Fat: 59g / Saturated Fat: 11g / Total Carbs: 2g

Dietary Fiber: 1g / Sugar: 1g / Protein: 13g / Sodium: 646mg

Vegan Curry Bowls
Preparation Time: 5 min - Cooking Time: 15 min - Servings: 4

Ingredients:

- 400 g Firm Tofu, sliced into bite-sized pieces
- 50 g Pineapple Chunks - 2 Roma Tomatoes, diced
- 1 small shallot, minced - 1 tbsp. Ginger-Garlic Paste
- 1 tbsp. Curry Powder - 1/3 cup Coconut Milk
- bunch of Cilantro, chopped - 2 tbsp. Olive Oil - Salt, to taste

Directions:

1. Heat olive oil in a non-stick pan.
2. Pan Fry tofu until brown on all sides. Set aside on paper towels to drain excess oil.
3. Pour off oil from the pan, leaving about a tablespoon.
4. Add shallots and ginger-garlic paste. Sautee until aromatic.
5. Add curry powder and roast briefly.
6. Add about half a cup of water and bring to a simmer.
7. Add tofu, pineapples, and tomatoes. Simmer until sufficiently reduced.
8. Add coconut milk and simmer until thick.
9. Simmer with salt to taste.

10. Garnish with chopped cilantro.

Nutrition: Calories: 272 / Fat: 21 g / Protein: 17 g / Carbs: 9 g

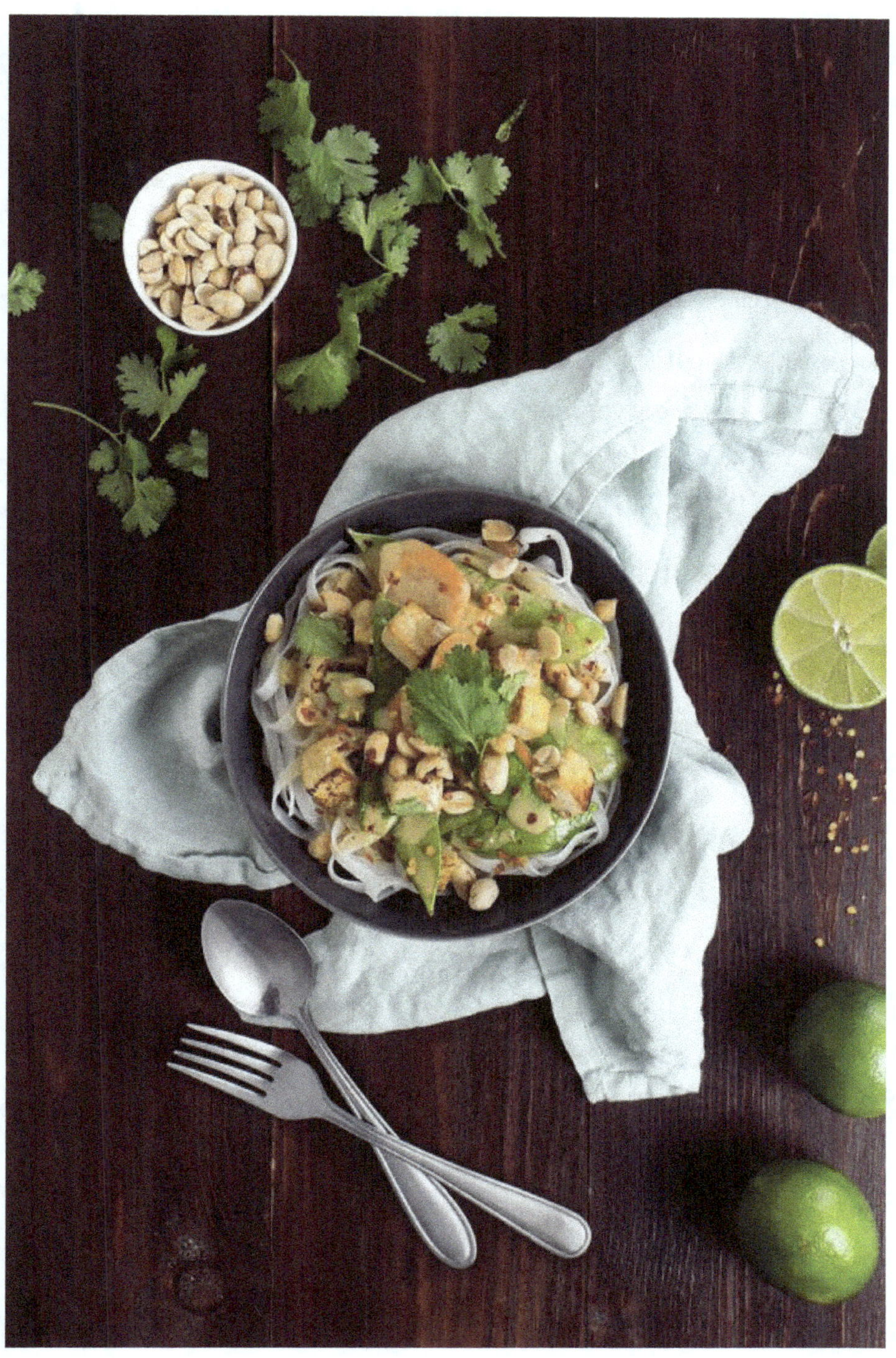

Smoky No-Meat Chili

Preparation Time: 10 min - Cooking Time: 20 min - Servings: 8

Ingredients:

- 400 g Cauliflower, trimmed and roughly chopped
- 400 g Quorn Mince - 400 g Crushed Tomatoes
- 2 cloves Garlic, minced - 1 small shallot, minced
- 1 tbsp. Vegan Worcestershire Sauce - 1 tbsp. Cumin Powder
- 1 tbsp. Paprika - 1 tsp Liquid Smoke
- 3 tbsp. Olive Oil - Salt and Pepper, to taste

Directions:

1. Put cauliflower in a food processor and pulse into a coarse texture.
2. Heat olive oil in a pot.
3. Sautee garlic and shallots until aromatic.
4. Add quorn and cauliflower. Sweat for a few minutes.
5. Add all remaining ingredients.
6. Cover the pot and simmer over low heat for 15-20 minutes.
7. Season with salt and pepper to taste.

8. Garnish with your choice of toppings.

Nutrition: Calories: 208 / Fat: 15 g / Protein: 10 g / Carbs: 10 g

Low-Carb Chinese Lo Mein
Preparation Time: 10 min - Cooking Time: 5 min - Servings: 6

Ingredients:

- 500 g Shirataki Noodles
- 150 g Shiitake Mushrooms, sliced
- 70 g Snow Peas - 70 g Baby Corn
- 100 g Red Bell Pepper, sliced
- 1 small shallot, minced
- 2 cloves Garlic, minced
- 1 tbsp. Peanut Oil
- 1 tbsp. White Wine Vinegar
- 2 tbsp. Low-Sodium Soy Sauce
- 2 tbsp. Sesame Oil - Salt and Pepper, to taste

Directions:

1. Prepare shirataki noodles according to package directions.
2. Heat peanut oil in a wok.
3. Add young corn and sauté for 1-2 minutes.
4. Add shiitake, snow peas, and red bell pepper — Stir-Fry for 1-2 minutes.
5. Add shallots and garlic. Sautee until aromatic.

6. Toss in prepared shirataki noodles together with the white wine vinegar, soy sauce, and sesame oil.

7. Season with salt and pepper as needed.

8. Serve hot.

Nutrition: Calories: 101 / Fat: 7 g / Protein: 2 g / Carbs: 9 g

www.ingramcontent.com/pod-product-compliance
Lightning Source LLC
Chambersburg PA
CBHW061003050726

47592CB00003B/1324